What athletes are saying about the Julstro Self-Treatments:

"Thank you. The treatment for the psoas exercise worked. I ran the Komen Race for the Cure this past Mother's Day, which was my first race. I completed it without a problem. Your book was one of the best running investments I could have made!"
Alexis

"Through Julie's methods and insights I have been able to keep my muscles looser and more durable. I'm better at avoiding injuries during training, I recover more quickly and smoothly after workouts, and my body is more comfortable and relaxed in general.

If I can convince just one other person to seek the benefits of Julstro — and enjoy the liberation of being able to achieve the same benefits on their own! — then that still won't be enough! I want EVERYBODY to know that they can take care of themselves, and how close they really are to being pain free."
Dave
Endurance Athlete

"I was beginning to think I would be walking Boston in April, but since I tried your shin splint treatment I feel 10 times better! It seems to do the trick - I could hardly walk before never mind run 26 miles! You're the greatest!"
Carmen

"I can't believe my abdominal cramps had anything to do with muscles in my legs!!! After many tests came out negative, I was losing hope I'd ever get rid of these cramps. I think this is going to be the one of the best books I have! I'm definitely going to spread the word about this!"
D.D. Massachusetts

"I just wanted you to know that the techniques I've learned from your website made it possible for me to complete my first half-Ironman this past April. I've been doing tri the past three years being constantly plague by one injury or the other. After finding your website I felt like I had been set free to really and finally enjoy this crazy sport. Thank-you so much for your invaluable service!"
Angela

Thanks to the calf-spasm-massage technique. After a painful 10 miler on Sunday, I thought I would have some significant downtime. After 2 days of massaging, went out and did 12 miles today! This may not work for everyone in every instance, but it is definitely worth a try!
Erich

"This book is a goldmine of information, extremely well organized, filled with the essential tools for excellence. Julie Donnelly offers a wealth of knowledge and experience on managing pain that can help athletes of all abilities achieve new levels of confidence and success - Highly recommended."JoAnn Dahlkoetter, Ph.D.

JoAnn Dahlkoetter, Ph.D., best-selling author of YOUR PERFORMING EDGE, is an internationally recognized sports psychologist, past winner of the San Francisco Marathon and 2nd in the Hawaii Ironman Triathlon.
650) 654-5500
3341 Brittan Ave., Suite #10
San Carlos, CA 94070-3435
Email: joann@sports-psych.com
Website: www.sports-psych.com

•••••••••••••••••••••••••••••••••••

"The Pain-Free Triathlete" is a must have for every multi-sport Athlete's library. Easy to understand, Julie's simple stated Self-treatment techniques are an integral part of my daily training regimen. This book will empower you to take better care of your body and spend more time doing what you love, "training and racing."

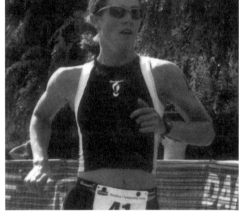

Rachel Sears
Professional Triathlete
Coach/Owner, Hypercat Racing
www.hypercatracing.com

The Self-Treatment techniques in this book have
helped thousands of athletes continue their sport
and be

Pain Free

The Pain-Free Triathlete

Julie Donnelly, LMT
and
Zev M. Cohen, MD

Makai Press, Nanuet, New York

The Pain-Free Triathlete

By: Julie Donnelly, LMT and Zev M. Cohen, MD

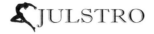

Published by:
Makai Press
79 Church Street
Nanuet, NY 10954
www.julstro.com
SAN: 2 5 5 - 4 1 6 X
Senior Editor: Jerry Trump
Book Layout: Textype
Illustrator: Jerry Trump
Library of Congress Control Number: 2003111450
Donnelly, Julie and Cohen, Zev
    The Pain-Free Triathlete
ISBN: 0-9741969-2-4
    1. Self-Help 2. Education & Teaching 3. Health & Fitness 4. Title

Legal Information

> The content of this manual is furnished for informational use only. It is not meant to replace medical care. WARNING: Many injuries and conditions are serious and require medical treatment by a qualified physician. Contact your physician prior to using the Julstro Techniques. Use of the treatments and/or programs in this book are done at the user's discretion.

Dedicated

To

The Pursuit of Health and Wellness

TABLE OF CONTENTS

ON THE COVER:
Rachael Sears (Bike)
Jerry Trump (Run)

FOREWORDS

Jerry Trump

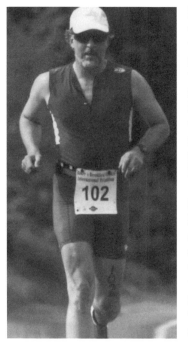

Have you ever had this happen to you – you spend years believing in a given "truth," or even doing something the same way for most of your life? Then "it" happens. It may be an event of some kind. Or someone you meet. It happens by accident. And then a whole new reality is upon you. You are faced with the realization that you have been completely blind. Out in the dark. Missing the boat.

So what am I talking about? I have been involved in athletics all my life. I can't remember a time when I wasn't on the Little League field, or doing whatever sport was in season. By the time I had reached college, I had been misfortunate enough to receive more than one "career ending" injury and multiple surgeries.

I still managed to play basketball at a NCAA division 1 level college, spending as much time in the care of sports trainers and doctors, as just about anybody. The point to this is that I've injured just about every part of my body at one time or another, playing one sport or another. Over the years, I've come to know the routine of treating sports related injuries quite well. Some of which I have overcome, and some of which I had come to the conclusion that I would have to live with. Over the last couple of years however, it meant not being able to train enough to compete in an Ironman distance triathlon. A dream that I had concluded would go unfulfilled.

I met Julie Donnelly completely by accident. I had given up on finding someone who could treat my Achilles Tendonitis with results. It would always re-occur with any lengthy training sessions. Julie sent me her book.

And that's when I had "it" happen to me. I found myself following directions and treating the mid-calf area of my leg, not my heel, (where all the pain was coming from). "How could that work?" From the time I had my first "booboo" the question was "where does it hurt?" and then the attention always focused on that area. And most certainly throughout my sports life, I don't remember one doctor fooling with a small spot on a muscle more that a foot away from my injury.

To keep this story short, here is the result. My $300.00 pair of prescription orthotics is in the closet, and I finished my first Ironman Triathlon in June of 2002. This is completely due to Julie's technique of treating repetitive strain injuries.

Julie Donnelly is not only an insightful and knowledgeable therapist, but she is also a teacher in the true sense of the word. I encourage you to take this book and use it as a guide to better health, better performance, and a better life. Don't be shocked to find that the pain in your shoulder just might be caused by a spasm in your back; and that you can treat it in a matter of minutes, not weeks.

Just remember that the recognized experts in the field used to think that the earth was flat.

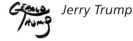 *Jerry Trump*

Paul Watson

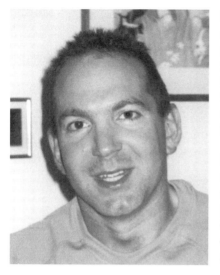

If you've ever had an injury that continually resurfaced after seemingly successful rehabilitation, or just one that refused to go away regardless of the various treatments, this book may very well hold the answers to your mysteries.

For nearly a decade I had dedicated hours of my daily schedule to rigorous training in pursuit of world-class physical conditioning necessary for highly competitive swimming, running, and rough-terrain racing events.

Over these years I had my share of strains, pulls, and bruises along the way but felt nearly invincible and confident nothing could keep me down.

However, I began injuring the area around my biceps-tendon on a regular basis, which routinely sidelined me from engaging in any meaningful swim training. Just when it was completely healed and I was confident it was 100%, sometimes for weeks, I would restrain it again. I thus began what turned out to be an exhaustive search of the healthcare industry for help. I saw orthopedists, massage therapists, neurologists, and chiropractors—in addition to having x-rays, MRI's, physical therapy, acupuncture, and ancient Chinese qui-gong performed on it—all to no avail. The "tendonitis" (as it was labeled) returned every time, shortly following the often-lengthy rehabilitation a "specialist" prescribed.

It took Julie Donnelly exactly two emails for her to correctly diagnose and solve this mystery. The problem: a shortening of the biceps muscle. The likely reason: all the aggressive swim training (hard intervals, weighted pull-ups, etc.). The solution: stretching. Hard to believe, isn't it? How could something so simple be so effective? Well, the advice and instruction not only worked for once, but also made perfect sense. The muscle was becoming shortened as a result of being in a prolonged state of contraction (2-4 hour swim workouts, 500 or so pull-ups over 90 minutes, etc.).

Not all of life's stories have a happy ending. Fortunately for me, this one does as I've seen these treatments work on me. If you are experiencing any training-related injuries, chances are great this book will help you successfully cure them. Follow the basic instructions she presents for any area that you have injured or have discomfort.

Finally this book can act as an exceptional preventative tool and I encourage you to read through it and take advantage of her knowledge.

Your training will surely benefit.

Paul Watson
Winner of 1999 "Beast of the East" competition

ACKNOWLEDGMENTS

Julie Donnelly, BS, LMT

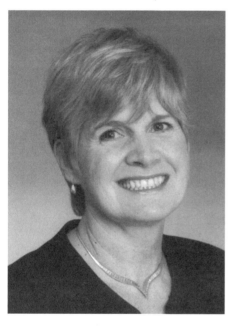

This series of Pain-Free books has become a true "Work in Progress"!

It all began in 1993 with some simple notes for my clients, many of whom were athletes and needed to learn how to immediately stop a pain that occurred during a training session, or a competition.

The next step, taken in 1999, was to gather together all the various notes I had written, and publish it as "How To Be Painless...A Beginner's Guide to the Self Treatment of Muscle Spasms". The models in this original book were real clients from my office, people of every age and body type, all of whom received benefit from the treatments. In fact, many of the treatments in the book were developed specifically for them!

In December 2001, Jerry Trump, an Ironman Triathlete with a severe Achilles tendonitis condition, found my book – and that was the beginning of this series. I'm glad to say that Jerry did successfully compete in the 2002 Utah Ironman Competition, and went on to finish a second Ironman event! We wish him Good Luck and Good Health with his continuing athletic efforts.

After Jerry learned how to successfully self-treat the source of his

Achilles Tendonitis, he convinced me to help athletes by going onto various forums, and that work became an eBook, "The Pain-Free Triathlete", and led to separate sport specific volumes. With this format, athletes will be able to focus on the muscles that they use the most. Jerry moved the entire Julstro Self-Treatment System to a new area that is exciting for me – working hand-in-hand with dedicated athletes through books, consultations, and Julstro Self Treatment Clinics both in gyms, and at major sporting events around the USA.

There are many people who have made this series of books become a reality, and I want to thank each person who has been a springboard for growth.

My wonderful family: my children Anne-Marie & Michael, their loving spouses Rob & Colleen, and the light of my life, my grandchildren: Meaghan, Ellen, Jack, Martin, Kate and Aidan. Thank you for listening to me as I endlessly went on & on "creating in my mind". You believed in me and loved me. I really appreciate how you inspired me.

I especially want to acknowledge my late friend, Beth, for teaching me that I was more than I believed. She started me on the road to an education, and was my constant cheering section. I know she sees this from her higher vantage point, and is smiling at me.

Zev Cohen, MD has been my supporter, my friend, and my toughest editor! He realized the value of what I was offering, long before the medical community would entertain the idea that muscles cause joint pain, and other chronic painful conditions. He invited me into his medical office to work with his patients, and showed me the perfect union between medicine and muscle therapy – I appreciate him immensely. The relationship has opened doors that I could only dream about – and we have both changed because of our mutual respect for each other.

His full participation in the self-treatment of Carpal Tunnel Syndrome was the catalyst to bringing this vital information out of the office, and into the homes of people around the world. We have proven that the pain and numbness associated with Carpal Tunnel Syndrome can be eliminated after just a few self-treatments! We have truly made a difference in the way this condition is being treated medically. We will continue our efforts until Carpal Tunnel Syndrome is no longer thought of as a debilitating condition.

Jerry Trump has been the catalyst for this stage in my growth - aside from inspiring me to write these books, Jerry's artistic ability is responsible for the beautiful graphics, and muscle drawings, that are used throughout all of the books, and for making the word "Julstro" become synonymous with relief from muscle &/or joint pain.

There were several others who have made this work become a reality. Special thanks go to:

- Paul Froehlich – for being one of the first people to believe in the Julstro Techniques, and for all the direction and hard work you did to support and inspire me. Thanks for helping to put "Julstro" into a video format, and into homes everywhere.

- Shawn Boom – we appreciate his excellent chapters on exercises specific to each book title.

- JoAnn Dahlkoetter, Ph.D. – For her chapter on paying attention to your body; often overlooked, but extremely important.

- Cassidy Phillips – For the work he has done that compliments everything we teach. We're so glad for all the input you have given us to help people learn even more techniques to heal themselves.

- Sue Kopac – for keeping the office running; finding lost objects, understanding my "multiple #1 priorities" and making sense out of them; doing her best to make the computer "user friendly"; and finally, for listening to me as I go into my excited visionary world!

- Our models: Rachel Sears, Jonathon Kent, Carin Phillips, Abbie Smith, Paul Watson, Greg Smith, Megan Bussart, Jerry Trump, Becky Thurn, and Bernie Casserly - all athletes who use the Julstro System on a daily basis, and have made the descriptions come alive. We appreciate their support!

Finally, speaking for both Dr. Cohen and myself, we are grateful to the real catalyst behind these books, our clients and patients, for the years of feedback that they have given us. There are too many to name, but each one was an important step in the development of these techniques.

Several of the original pictures and stories have been transferred over from my first book, and athletes I've worked with online have sent testimonials and photos to be included into the new books. While our models, and the athletes who gave testimonials, aren't famous to the world, their stories are real – and without them these books would not exist.

My life has been blessed by all of the people I have just mentioned, and so many others. I hope you enjoy the books, and that the self-treatments bring you the benefits that others have experienced.

Yours in Health,

Julie

Julie Donnelly

Zev M. Cohen, M.D.

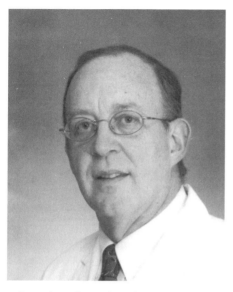

"When did you decide to become a doctor?" is a question I am often asked. My answer is always the same. It probably started when I was an infant in my mother's arms. She would show me off to her friends and say, "this is my son, he's going to be a doctor!"

Well, maybe that's not exactly how it happened. What is certain is the love and devotion my parents showed me while I was growing up. Not only did they teach me the importance of a good education, but also they instilled in me the values of honesty, caring, love, charity and compassion. Tools as necessary as a stethoscope for the daily practice of medicine.

My father taught me that I could do anything, if I try hard enough, and my mother taught me to think for myself and not follow the crowd. I am who I am because of who they are!

My gratitude to my loving parents goes beyond words. The feelings that I have, and carry with me every day of my life, are precious and for that I am forever grateful.

Not many years ago I was practicing medicine in a busy Internal Medicine office. I practiced by "the book", the way I had been taught in my medical school and residency training. But in my heart I knew there was a lot more to the practice of medicine. Medical textbooks didn't have all the answers!

I met Julie Donnelly at a Charity Health Fair; our immediate connection was, I feel, divinely inspired. She opened my mind to an area of medicine that is glaringly missing from medical training: the area of treating muscles to relieve many types of acute and chronic conditions. This new understanding has dramatically changed the way I treat patients on a daily basis.

Together, we have been able to restore many people to good health, allowing people to be pain free – and many times we have rescued people from "the knife". Julie's techniques of treating muscles, called the Julstro System, has so effectively been able to treat conditions such as Carpal Tunnel syndrome, that surgery has been cancelled on countless occasions. Julie, as the quintessential teacher, has taught thousands of patients how to treat themselves. Not only are they pain free when they leave my office, but they are equipped with the knowledge of how to treat their condition, should it return. Her tireless energy, strong focus, and never-ending enthusiasm are what keep both the Carpal Tunnel Treatment Center, and Julstro Muscular Therapy Center, going strong. I can't thank her enough.

My family, friends, and office staff, are all collectively a part of this book. I have always considered us a team – each member of the team vitally important.

And, of course, I must thank the Creator of our wonderful universe – whose Pure and Good Energy is what keeps us all going!

Zev M. Cohen, MD

INTRODUCTION

You have decided that you need to take an important aspect of your well being into your own hands – wise move!

Years of experience with thousands of individuals; athletes, "weekend warriors" and "couch potatoes", has proven to us that muscle spasms are a primary cause of muscle pains and joint pains. We have seen people run from one doctor to another to get an answer – and still be in pain. They have gone to physical therapy, massage therapy, chiropractic, and taken medication by the truckload, and still the pain persists. Why?

The answer will become crystal clear as you read this book. Muscle spasms are the major culprit to the vast majority of joint and muscle pains.

Why You Need This Book

Every day you do the same movements over and over. They may be at work, or while you are relaxing. Exercise will certainly stress your body, pushing it beyond its limits! It also causes the muscles to suffer from repetitive strain injury, causing pain, often severe pain that prevents you from living your life as you choose.

When joint pain develops you are told to use RICE – "Rest, Ice, Compression and Elevation". But – YOU DON"T WANT TO REST! Exercise is your lifeblood; it is what makes you thrive. That is why we wrote *The Pain-Free Triathlete* – to keep you moving and pain-free!

What To Do If Your Area of Pain Is Not In This Book

The Pain-Free Triathlete grew from simple beginnings of working with clients in our office and in a book called *How To Be Pain-less…A Beginner's Guide To The Self Treatment of Muscle Spasms.*

Athletes kept asking about problems that weren't in the original book, and eventually an eBook was written in 2002. Again, athletes were continuously asking about situations that weren't in *The Pain-Free Triathlete eBook,* and a newsletter was developed to share the new treatments as they developed.

We added the treatments from the newsletters while writing this book. Even before the book went to the printer more new treatments were developed because of work we are doing with endurance and professional athletes who are getting injured in their quest for personal achievement. We have come to realize that this book will never be complete – new techniques will continue to be designed to help athletes who need our assistance.

If you have a pain that isn't covered by this book, email us at: Julie@julstro.com. We'll work together to find your answer, and that will be the material for the next revision of *The Pain-Free Triathlete.*

The good news is, in the vast majority of cases we are able to find the spasm that is causing your problem, even if it is a long-standing problem. Once we find the cause, it's easy to work out the technique necessary to eliminate that spasm, giving you relief.

We look forward to hearing from you!

How this Book is Organized

The Pain-Free Triathlete is divided into four parts:

Part I – Healthy Advice for Endurance Athletes
Part II – All You'll Ever Need to Know About Muscles and Joints
Part III – The Julstro Treatments
Part IV –Trigger Point / Muscle Charts and Glossaries

Part I – Healthy Advice for Endurance Athletes – Listening to the Wisdom of the Body

Written by JoAnn Dahlkoetter, Ph.D., best-selling author of YOUR PERFORMING EDGE. JoAnn is an internationally recognized sports psychologist, past winner of the San Francisco Marathon and 2nd place finisher in the Hawaii Ironman Triathlon World Championship.

Part II – All You'll Ever Need to Know About Muscles and Joints

Read Part II thoroughly to understand the "why" and "how" of muscles. They are the cause of your pain, and knowing how they work will enable you to treat them properly and quickly.

Chapter 1, Our Magnificent Muscles
In this chapter you will receive the basics of muscle movement and why muscles will shorten. This is the key to the entire problem and can't be overlooked.

Chapter 2, The Basics: How a Joint Moves
This chapter builds on Chapter 1 information and answers many questions.

Chapter 3, Avoiding Needless Surgery: Backs, Knees, and Carpal Tunnel Syndrome
In this chapter we examine why muscles have been ignored when searching for the answer to joint and muscle pain. It takes a general look at conditions that can be easily reversed by simply finding and treating the muscle spasms, and then stretching the muscle back to its proper length. This chapter shows why muscles cause conditions that are typically not considered to be a muscular problem, such as carpal tunnel syndrome, rotator cuff, knee pain, and how you can stop it immediately.

Chapter 4, Prevent Injuries Through Proper Exercise
This chapter introduces a vital key to being a Triathlete and staying pain-free. Avoiding problems in the first place should be your personal goal. This chapter focuses on an Introduction to Physiology of Exercise and is written by Shawn Boom. An Ironman Triathlete himself, Shawn is an Exercise Physiologist and Personal Fitness Trainer for elite athletes.

Chapter 5, The Core Workouts for Fast Triathletes
This chapter offers you a training program that is well balanced and geared to preventing injuries while still

maximizing your training program. This chapter is a natural "fit" in *The Pain-Free Triathlete* and completes the process of learning how to exercise at your optimum level – and stay well!

Chapter 6, The Julstro™ Method of Self-treatment

A complete explanation of the Julstro System is covered in this chapter. These will be your everyday "tools" to keep your muscles and joints healthy.

Chapter 7, The Trigger Point Charts

Trigger points are introduced, along with charts that are designed to help you locate the source of your pain. This chapter is the core of *The Pain–Free Triathlete* and is required reading to ensure that you use this book properly as a resource guide.

Part III – The Julstro Treatments

The chapters that make up this section of the book combine the areas shown in the trigger point charts with the Julstro self-treatments. Clear, easy-to-read text is complimented with photographs to help you to find and treat the spasms that are causing you pain. Each body part is individually covered.

Part IV –Trigger Point / Muscle Charts and Glossaries

On the trigger point charts you locate where you are feeling the pain – and you will find where the true source of that pain can be found. The spasm is often far from the area of discomfort, in fact, it may even be on the opposite side of your body!

The logic is simple to follow when using these charts. After you locate the area of pain on the referenced Trigger Point Chart, simply look up the muscle that is listed in the Table of Contents. You will be directed to the treatment for that muscle.

The muscle charts show you the details of the muscle connections, which help you to understand why you can feel pain in area distant from the spasm.

Where to Go From Here

Take a minute to glance through the book, getting comfortable with what's inside. Read Part One thoroughly, then start to relieve the pains that are holding you down.

Is it possible to be a triathlete, and be pain-free?

YOU BET IT IS!!

PART I: HEALTHY ADVICE FOR ENDURANCE ATHLETES – LISTENING TO THE WISDOM OF THE BODY

By JoAnn Dahlkoetter, Ph.D.

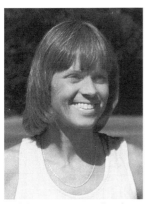

Learn to hear the whispers of the body and mind before they have to shout

An athlete came into my office a month ago complaining that, "Whenever an important race comes up something goes wrong, either mentally or physically. I can't seem to pull it all together when it really counts. I seem to be counterproductive, self-defeating, and continually sabotaging myself." I hear this type of complaint from athletes across the board, regardless of what sport or what level of play. For example, running can be such a challenging sport that requires so many bones, muscles, and connective tissue to work well together, it's easy to misjudge the body's limits and create an injury.

In team sports we're often taught by coaches to not pay too much attention to aches and pains. We are told: "Don't be a wimp – just get through the work out. We have a race this Sunday." So we often ignore the subtle symptoms. We prod on, making sure we complete our designated weekly mileage, doing a small amount of tissue damage each day, until our body screams for attention. Once an injury sets in, the healing and recovery then takes much longer than if we had learned to pay attention each day.

Sports Car Mentality

The body in fact has critical information for us. We need only to listen carefully, sense its soft messages, and follow its direction regularly. We need to first check in with our bodies before blindly moving ahead with our training plan. Indeed, **to train consistently and to stay healthy, we need to treat and care for our bodies like a finely tuned sports car.**

Over the next month I worked with the athlete described above. I showed him a technique involving listening and dialoguing where he learned to tune in to his body and mind with a sense of compassion and curiosity. In fact he launched into a journey that led to profound and lasting change in his running, which then carried over to the rest of his life. I have used this dialoguing technique successfully with so many athletes that it is well worth incorporating into your training plans. The process does not take extra time, only a greater awareness during the time you are training.

What I'm proposing here is a body-oriented process of awareness and healing. You can learn a method of sensing how you feel – physically and mentally. Then you can have a dialogue with your feelings and sensations where **you** do most of the **listening.** Athletes tend to be action-oriented, driven, and goal-directed. **They are accustomed to actively telling their bodies what to do - most of the time not so tactfully.**

You may say to yourself: "Pick up the pace, you slug, your shoulders are too stiff, why aren't you catching that guy in front of you?" What do you do when an uncomfortable feeling develops in your body (e.g. calf cramping or knee aching)? The typical reaction is to try to over-ride it. Perhaps you yell at it a bit: "Why does this stupid pain have to come on right now, when I've got 13 miles to go in the marathon?" Or you might beat yourself up mentally: "If only I had trained harder, my knee wouldn't freeze up like this."

Becoming Quiet and Listening

What does not occur to most athletes is to become quiet and to listen to the body's sensations. The key to preventing injury is to let your body give you this crucial feedback, especially while warming up for your regular workouts. Then you can take in and respect its wisdom before deciding on your course of action.

When you let the body speak, you are allowing yourself to be open to the depth and richness of your whole self – body, mind, and spirit. Once you pay attention to a sensation (e.g. tension or pain), it is more likely to release, and let you go on with your training in a more clear, and focused way. You'll also gain a better sense of what you need to do, if anything, to help the body function more efficiently (e.g. alter your posture, training form, breathing, etc.). Often we don't need to change anything at all. The body can heal and correct itself. **Awareness alone can often take care of the problem.**

Have you ever wondered during workout, "Am I doing the right thing for my body today? Should I be going this far, or this fast when I'm just returning from an injury? Is this workout helping to strengthen that area, or is it further aggravating the tendons that are still weak and vulnerable? Am I ready to take my training to the next level, or should I be conservative and stay with the same workouts for another week?" Regular listening and dialoguing with the body, as I will describe below, can fully answer all these questions, and give you a strong sense that you are doing the right thing.

Consulting With Your Body

It is now well accepted that we can confer with our bodies to assess if we are eating the proper food and if we are getting enough sleep. We understand that our bodies know what it feels like to be in good health, and what it's like when we're on the edge of a cold or flu, or injury. We know the positive sensations of having energy to spare and being very focused. We also know when we've let ourselves become way too tired or let our bodies get torn down.

Indeed, **we understand how to recognize the extreme states, but what about the subtle stages in between?** With arduous training and regularly challenging the muscles and tissues to work harder, we are continually tearing the body down. And don't forget, the mind is also challenged and needs recovery. This repair and healing process is going on constantly, for both the body and mind. The question is what are you doing to be more aware, and to facilitate that healing process?

Our bodies are wise in many ways beyond what is acknowledged by the average person. They can show us the path to optimal health and fitness if we so choose. Our bodies carry knowledge not only about how we are training, but how we are treating ourselves, what we value and believe, how we have been hurt emotionally, and how we are living our lives. Have you ever noticed when you think about that coach or parent who mistreated you, the pain in your neck or shoulder gets worse? Our bodies know which people are good for us to train with and which ones deplete and degrade us. And our physical selves know the best path to move up to the next level in our performance.

Below I have described a technique of tuning in and listening to the body in a caring, non-judgmental way that can save you months of time being on the injured list. Using this technique of listening and dialoguing can become a window into this expansive domain of knowledge that is accessible through the body. This type of work allows you to hear the soft warnings of the body and mind before they have to scream for attention. Then you'll be on your way to remaining healthy throughout the year.

Benefits of Listening to the Body

What kinds of problems best lend themselves to this sort of technique?

- Athletes who are training hard but feel stuck can use this listening technique to get their training moving again. You may be wondering: "I keep doing the same workouts, but the progress isn't there. There's something I'm not understanding about my body and my training."

- Some athletes may need to work on a problem with an addiction (e.g. overeating, drinking, caffeine, drugs). This technique can help release you from the power of your addiction by allowing you to listen carefully to the part of you that is responsible for the addictive behavior, and gain its cooperation.

- Athletes who have difficult or overwhelming feelings can learn to have a better relationship with their emotions. Strong feelings (anger, fear, sadness) can sometimes wash over us like ocean waves, and they can interrupt effective training. However, these emotions are there for a reason. They have an important message to convey. They bring back an important part of our wholeness. We need to learn to listen to their story without becoming overwhelmed. With this technique, you can begin to have a comfortable relationship with strong feelings, and acknowledge them without being drowned by them.

- Competitive athletes often have a highly critical side that makes training less enjoyable. You may want to quiet your critical side and enhance self-acceptance. With practice, you can turn your inner critic into an ally and supporter. Once you accept all parts of yourself (e.g. even the part that sometimes gets injured) this will allow deeper and more meaningful improvement in your training.

Creating an Atmosphere of Trust

Before beginning the work of listening to the body, we need to first establish a safe, trusting environment for communication. Imagine for a moment that you are walking along a trail, and you notice a small bashful animal peeking out from behind a tree. The animal is not a danger to you, but you would like to help it feel safe and relax around you. How would you accomplish this? What atmosphere would you like to create? You certainly would not run toward it shouting. You would probably be still and patient, or move very slowly and gently. You would be interested in it, watching carefully for signs that it feels comfortable around you. You would notice when it might be all right to move in a little closer.

The technique of dialoguing with your body described below is a process of listening to something inside yourself that wants to communicate with you. Just like getting to know the shy animal, your body may first need to establish that you are trustworthy, that you have created a safe place for it to deliver its message. So you need to create a safe, non-judgmental environment to do this work. Now you're ready to try this exercise.

Awareness Exercise #1 – Being in touch with your Body:

Take a moment and notice what you are feeling right now in your body or mind. If you are working out, notice if you have any nagging pain. Is it possible to simply let the feeling be there without trying to change it? Just notice how you are in this moment and say: "Yes, this is how I feel". Or say to the uncomfortable sensation: "Yes, I know you're there". You may have a tendency to judge your body as soon as you notice any discomfort and say, "I shouldn't be feeling this way". Or you may try to analyze your body pain saying: "Why do I always feel this way? Why doesn't my body perform like I want it to?" None of these ways are effective in helping the situation. This usually creates more body tension and discomfort.

However, when you allow your bodily sensations to be as they are and just acknowledge them, then they can change for the better on their own. When they are allowed just to be, they can settle down to have a conversation with you, and that conversation leads to positive change. You can really tune in and understand what your symptoms are telling you.

I utilized this exercise with one of my athlete clients who was experiencing hamstring pain while training for an ice dancing competition. After acknowledging the sensation she noticed an immediate sense of physical relief. She said: "The sensation is still there, but it's no longer painful. Now that it has my attention, it doesn't need to hurt and nag at me anymore."

Awareness Exercise #2 – Dialoguing with your Body:

Once you've established an area of your body that you would like to work on, you can begin a dialogue. Ask yourself: "What bodily sensation am I most aware of? What part needs my attention?" Once you identify a certain area, then ask yourself: "What exactly does it feel like?" Find the right words to describe it. Make sure you have the best words to fully articulate how it feels (e.g. tight shoulders, heavy feet, mind racing, etc.) You can write these thoughts down in a journal later. Next, gently acknowledge its presence. You could say, for instance: "Yes, I know you're there." Rather than fighting with the body as we often do, saying, "Oh God, there's that darn knee pain again", this time you can simply notice the sensation with a quiet curiosity, and begin to learn about it. Then just notice what happens. Become aware of any change in the sensation.

Now you can begin asking that part of the body what it needs. Or you can ask: "What needs to happen next for it to get better?" You can learn, for instance, if it just needs your quiet company? Does it need more care and attention? Does it need some special treatment?

Next you could **ask your body to show you how "completely healed" would feel.** How would it feel to have the problem cleared up, resolved satisfactorily. The body knows now how it would feel to have the situation resolved, even though your analytical mind may have no idea how that could happen. Ask your body to show you by beginning to feel that way right now. That kind of suggestion helps create an opening for new ways of being and perhaps healthier ways of treating your body.

The body's solutions are infinitely better, more creative, and healthier than anything your logical mind can dream up. You may feel stuck, but your body isn't. Once you begin to listen, understand, and dialogue with your body, it will show you its ageless wisdom. It will let you in on its critical secrets for staying healthy and moving forward with your training. You can then train more consistently and remain healthy throughout the year. You'll gain a new level of sensitivity to the body that can take you to new performance highs.

JoAnn Dahlkoetter, Ph.D., author of YOUR PERFORMING EDGE, is an internationally recognized sports psychologist, past winner of the San Francisco Marathon and 2nd in the Hawaii Ironman Triathlon. To see her NEW BOOK and VISUALIZATION CD, visit www.YourPerformingEdge.com, or call 650- 654-5500. Dr. Dahlkoetter provides coaching by phone for optimal mind-body performance. For a FREE NEWSLETTER with valuable training tips and articles, Email: joann@YourPerformingEdge.com.

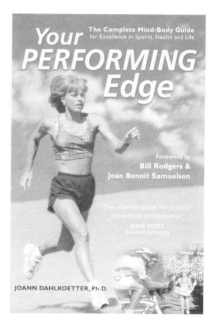

PART II: ALL YOU'LL EVER NEED TO KNOW ABOUT MUSCLES AND JOINTS

CHAPTER 1

Our Magnificent Muscles

Zev M. Cohen, MD

Our muscles comprise the largest part of our body. Indeed, they are the largest single organ of the body, and make up the bulk of its weight. All together, humans have about 300 paired-muscles, totaling approximately 600 muscles.

Each muscle, or muscle group, has its unique function. Some muscles work alone, others work together in unison. The amount of movements we possess, as a result of the combination of muscle fibers being utilized, are unlimited. Observe your hand and wrist, and the number of ways it moves, turns, twists, and so on. Despite all this movement, each muscle has only one function, i.e.: to contract or relax. As one muscle group contracts (shortens), an opposing muscle group relaxes (lengthens).

It's that simple...or is it?

An absolutely perfect symphony of movements must take place for each step we take. When you ate breakfast this morning, the muscles responsible for chewing had to contract, and relax, thousands upon thousands of times! In fact, to continue our example of breakfast, let's take a closer look at what was involved.

You used the muscles of your foot and toes, ankles, legs, thighs, and back, to go to the table and sit down. The muscles of your eyes, neck, shoulders, chest, arms, wrists, hand, and fingers were all in motion. And lastly, of course the muscles of the face, which are responsible for chewing and swallowing, were working constantly.

And what's most amazing is we didn't give it a single thought – it all "sort of" took place naturally!

The muscles of the human body are in use 24 hours a day, 7 days a week, 365 days a year. Despite this enormous amount of use, most of us spend little, or no, time caring for our muscles. Obviously, with such extensive and continued use, we must experience "wear and tear". In medical terms, this is known as Repetitive Strain Injury (RSI).

Let's face it; we are all creatures of habit. Which means we tend to do the same things in the same way, over and over again. The way I brushed my teeth this morning was exactly the same way I brushed them before bedtime. That goes for yesterday, the day before, and probably the last 10-20 years. The way we sit, stand, walk, drive, read a book, exercise, work at a computer – and any other movement – are ali-important elements to the condition of our muscles.

Whether you are a homemaker or a construction worker... a typist or an interstate trucker... a musician or an electrician...the stress and strain placed on your muscles, each and every day, is enormous!

Repetitive Strain Injuries, or "wear and tear", tend to occur most often when muscles are used repeatedly, the more strength used, the more stress is placed on the muscle. However, you do not need to be moving to be using a muscle!

While quietly sitting and reading a book, although seeming relaxed, the muscles of the fingers, hands, and arm are all in use. The same goes for the neck and back muscles. It's ironic, isn't it, that you can be the victim of Repetitive Strain Injury while quietly sitting in your easy chair, reading a book! In fact, sitting is a very common cause of low back pain, because it contracts a muscle called the psoas. The more force exerted, the longer the time the muscle group is in use, and the less time spent on relaxing, and stretching, are all important factors to muscle injury.

Sometimes it's obvious: you mowed the lawn or shoveled snow from the walk, or started an aerobics class, and the next day you are sore, or maybe you had low back pain the day after lifting your child. These are simple cause and effect injuries. However, very often it is much less obvious - a contracted muscle in the neck or chest might cause pain and discomfort to the wrist and hand, which are the symptoms of carpal tunnel syndrome, but there isn't any pain in the neck or chest. This is known as "referred pain".

In the 1960's, Janet Travell, MD, conducted research that proved that muscle spasms caused pain to be felt in areas far from the spasm. She called the spasms "Trigger Points". Muscles often cause many–previously not well-understood– illnesses, such as: fibromyalgia, tinnitis (ringing in the ears), headaches, TMJ (jaw pain), many arthritic conditions, joint pains, tennis elbow, sciatica, and carpal tunnel syndrome!

To understand why a muscle causes pain, it is necessary to have a basic understanding of the anatomy of muscles. A muscle has two ends; at each end there is a covering of connective tissue called a tendon. Each tendon connects to a bone, usually crossing a joint. When a muscle contracts, one bone remains stationary and forms a fixed point, the other end pulls the bone to make the joint move.

For example, let's look at the flexor muscle group, the thick muscles on the underside of your forearm. One end of the flexor muscles attaches to the arm near the inside of your elbow. The other end inserts onto your wrist, hand and fingers. When the flexors are relaxed your hand is open. When the flexors contract, it shortens and you can see, or feel, the muscle thicken your forearm. The shortening of the flexor cause your hand to curl into a fist, and your fist to move toward your arm.

The basic unit of a muscle is a single fiber. These individual fibers are grouped together to form a bundle of muscles. Each individual muscle fiber operates according to the "all or nothing" principle. This means that when the muscle fiber is stimulated, it will contract with all its force, it will not stop in the middle of the contraction. There is no middle of the road with a muscle; it is all – or nothing!

In reality, and under certain adverse conditions, muscle fibers might contract and remain "stuck" in the contracted position. This may cause an acute pain, such as a muscle spasm, or a cramp, which can be severe.

Usually, however, the results of shortened muscle fibers are more subtle. For example, shortened muscles might be the cause of someone's "hunch back", chronic headache, or carpal tunnel syndrome!

CHAPTER 2

The Basics: How a Joint Moves and Other Interesting Info

A muscle crossing over a joint gives that joint the ability to move. Movement of a joint is a two-step process: one muscle must contract and shorten while the opposing muscle must relax and lengthen.

When a spasm occurs in the muscle, the pain is usually felt at the insertion of the muscle (the place where the muscle attaches to the bone), which is at the joint. In the case of the biceps, the insertion is on the inside of your elbow on the lower portion of your arm, while the insertion of the triceps is just below the point of your elbow, so spasms in either of these muscles will most likely cause elbow pain.

While the contract/stretch rule is the process of every muscle throughout the body, for demonstration purposes we will show how the biceps muscle (A) and the triceps (B) work together.

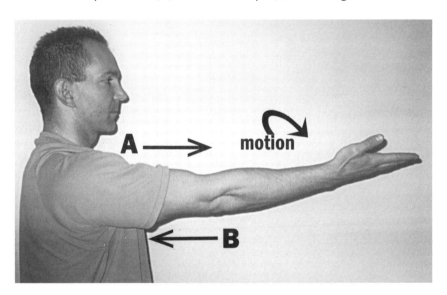

To open your arm, the biceps must stretch (A) and the triceps must contract/shorten (B).

When the biceps contract (A) and the triceps stretch (B) the arm bends at the elbow.

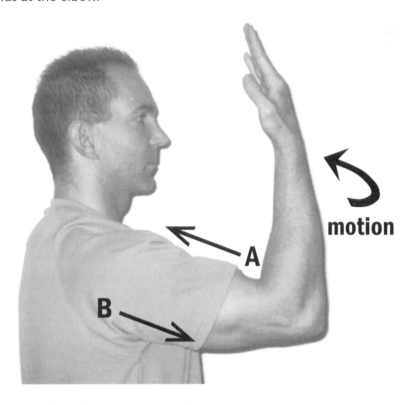

In order to be able to completely bend or straighten the arm, these muscles must both be able to contract and stretch fully. If, for example, the biceps contract and the triceps do not stretch, the restricted triceps will stop the movement and you will not be able to fully bend your arm.

The ankle joint is controlled by several muscles.

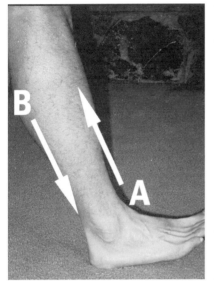

When the tibialis anterior (A) contracts it lifts your toes from the ground.

Meanwhile the calf muscles and Achilles tendon (B) must stretch.

In your calf you have two primary muscles with the Latin names: gastrocneimus (commonly called "gastroc"), and soleus. The "gastroc", originates above the knee, so it also assists at bending your knee; the soleus originates in the middle of the calf. They both go into the tendon in the back of your ankle, called the Achilles tendon, and then continue on to insert on the back of your heel.

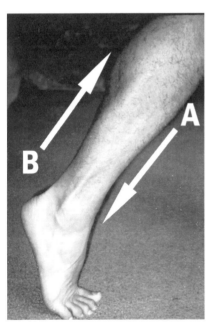

When the calf muscles are contracted they pull on the Achilles tendon, which then pulls on the heel, allowing you to "push off" with your toes (B). To make this movement the tibialis anterior must stretch (A).

Under the primary calf muscles, there are also lesser known muscles which do not go into the Achilles tendon. These include the tibialis posterior, flexor digitorum longus and flexor hallucis longus. A spasm will cause pain in this area, making one think there is a problem with the Achilles tendon.

A muscle spasm, or contracted muscle, will cause pain at the insertion point of the muscle. This is known as referred pain. We use the following example to clearly illustrate this situation: if you pull your hair at the end, it hurts at the scalp where it inserts. It is the same with muscles. If you contract (pull) the bulk of the muscle (known as the belly of the muscle), it will hurt where the muscle inserts into the bone. When your calf muscles are contracted, they may hurt directly on the muscle. However, since it is pulling on the insertion, your heel may hurt – even when you aren't feeling anything in the calf!

Another phenomenon attests to the wisdom of the body. As the muscle is pulling the tendon away from the bone, the body sends bone cells to secure the attachment. As these bone cells collect, you get what is called a "spur", or a bump of bone. This is frequently seen at the heel and at the shoulder. To try to break down the spur without releasing the muscle tightness first is fruitless. The body's intelligence will simply send more bone cells to secure the tendon.

Stretching is vital to the movements of joints. A stretch works best when it is only done to the degree that it feels good, (you'll always know where that is), and is held for one full minute. We have seen people exercise – some to excess – but they rarely stretch sufficiently.

That is what this book is all about: using the Julstro System to release the tight spasms and contractions, and stretch your muscles. When you release a spasm you are also lengthening the muscle – it's like untying a knot and the rope gets longer.

Sprains Affect on Muscles

When you sprain a joint, for example the ankle, the muscles are suddenly overstretched, and then quickly released, causing multiple spasms to form in the muscle. Since a muscle is normally held in perfect tension, from the origination to the insertion, these spasms will cause a stress to be placed on the insertion point of the muscle at the joint, causing pain that will not cease until the spasms are released.

A sprain at any joint requires treatment of the spasms found in each muscle that crosses that joint. After the spasms are treated stretching will relieve the tension on the joint.

Broken Bones Effect on Muscles

When the bone breaks the muscle suddenly contracts totally. As the bone is set the muscle is pulled into place, but rarely are the muscle spasms treated to bring the fibers back to their correct length.

This results in the bone being strained by the multiple spasms that have formed during the sudden contraction. We have seen clients who have experienced pain for years after a fracture, even though the bone has healed perfectly. As soon as the muscle spasms are treated the pressure is removed from the bone, and pain is eliminated.

CHAPTER 3

Avoiding Needless Surgeries!

Through the years we have had countless numbers of clients come to our offices with severe joint pain. Many times they had already been thru a wide assortment of therapies without finding relief, and had then been scheduled to have surgery. On many occasions they didn't even come to us about the joint problem, they were there for other reasons and just "happened to mention it" to one of us. As you read this book you will find several examples of people who were heading for needless surgery – and were "spared the knife" by using the Julstro method of deep muscle therapy.

Of course, there are times when only surgery will help. When a tendon or ligament has been severed, only re-attaching the pieces will give pain relief and return mobility.

When you read Chapter 1, Our Magnificent Muscles, you gained an understanding of how muscles cause joint pain; therefore, we will only include a brief explanation here. Muscles insert at a joint, and when the muscle contracts the joint moves. However, when the muscle is in spasm it continues to contract, even when you are trying to move the joint in a different direction. Just as pulling your hair will cause you pain where it inserts at the scalp, so does pulling a tight muscle cause pain where it inserts at the joint. In his book "What You Don't Know Can Hurt You…Seven Important Facts about Carpal Tunnel Syndrome", Dr. Cohen has explained: "medical doctors aren't trained in how pain is caused by muscles. This is a major gap in understanding the body, and in pain management."

This is the case whether it is the quadriceps muscles that inserts at the knee, the calf muscles that insert at the Achilles tendon and the heel, the triceps muscle that inserts into the elbow; or any of the muscles of the forearm that insert into the wrist and hand. There have been innumerable surgeries done on joints that could have been avoided if only the muscles had been treated and lengthened.

When the muscles of the body cross over a nerve, such as the sciatic nerve in the buttocks, a spasm in the muscle will cause pain and numbness to be felt far from the spasm. In the case of the sciatic nerve the pain/numbness is felt in the hip, hamstrings, calf and arch of the foot.

While the problem occurs throughout the entire body, this is clearly understood by using wrist pain as an example. When a person is having pain in the hand and wrist, and numbness in the fingers, he may be misdiagnosed as having "carpal tunnel syndrome". This problem of misdiagnosis warrants further explanation.

Carpal Tunnel Syndrome is the #1 repetitive strain injury (RSI) in the USA, accounting for an estimated 400,000 carpal tunnel release surgeries in 2001. Tragically, many of these surgeries could easily have been avoided!

As we mentioned earlier, using the hair-pulling example, if you pull your hair your scalp will hurt. Don't "fix the scalp, let go of the hair. Carpal tunnel is exactly the same situation. Don't operate on the tunnel, simply let go of the muscles that are causing a strain at the tunnel – or at any point along the length of the median nerve.

Carpal Tunnel Syndrome occurs when the nerve in the wrist and hand (called the median nerve) becomes entrapped. The fact is, if the median nerve is entrapped anywhere along its entire length, one may experience wrist/hand pain and numbness. This is the vital piece that is being overlooked by most practitioners.

Since 95% of the median nerve is not in the carpal tunnel, it is safe to surmise that 95% of the potential source of the pain and numbness is not coming from within the tunnel. Therefore 95% of the surgery is unnecessary – *that would total 380,000 needless surgeries in 2001!*

The same can be said for knee surgery, low back surgery, and ankles.... the list goes on! Muscles are a serious missing piece in the pre-surgical treatment process. In the chapter on the shoulder, you will read that a spasm in the infraspinatus muscle will give the same symptoms as bursitis of the shoulder, and can also mimic the pain of a torn rotator cuff; the chapter on the leg shows how a spasm in the quadriceps will cause searing pain to be felt in the knee. However, surgery is NOT the answer – only releasing the muscle spasms will relieve the pain!

In order to stop the pain in your hand, and numbness in your fingers, to continue working and enjoying your life to the fullest, and to avoid potential surgery, it is important to understand the anatomy of the Carpal Tunnel. We suggest you visit our website (www.julstro.com) so you may view the graphics demonstrating each step of this explanation.

There are 8 small bones in the wrist called the "carpal bones". These bones form the base of the carpal tunnel. A ligament called the Flexor Retinaculum, also known as the Transverse Carpal Ligament, forms the roof of the tunnel, commonly called "the bridge". Lay the back of your hand on a table, and look at this graphic.

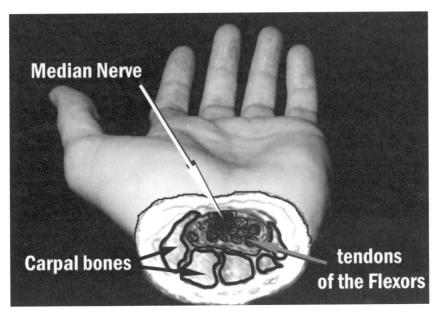

Through the small carpal tunnel passes the nine flexor tendons, along with the median nerve.

Any pressure exerted onto this area will squeeze the median nerve and cause pain and numbness to the hand and wrist.

For example: repetitive wrist or hand motions, such as working at a computer terminal, playing a musical instrument, sports, or even knitting, will cause swelling in the carpal tunnel.

To complicate things, the median nerve, which starts in the neck and travels down the arm to the wrist and hand, can become entrapped anywhere along its path by any of the muscles that cross over it. A pinched nerve in the neck, or anywhere along the path of the median nerve, may cause you to have pain in your hand. A simple analogy will demonstrate this point: A telephone line a few blocks away, when knocked down after a storm, may cause static on your telephone. This concept is exactly what happens when the median nerve is pressed on, or irritated anywhere along its entire path, a static message is sent to the muscle.

If you have access to a computer you can click on http://www.aboutcts.com/median_nerve.html to view the median nerve. This is the nerve that will cause pain and numbness to be felt in the chest, the upper back, the entire arm and also the hand.

The first muscle that may impact on the median nerve is the scalenes, which originate on your cervical (neck) vertebrae and insert onto the first rib.

When the scalenes are contracted by a spasm, they put pressure directly onto a bundle of nerves called the brachial plexus. This causes a multitude of problems, including numbness in the thumb and first two fingers.

The median nerve continues through the chest, arm and into the hand. Each of the following links will describe another part of the condition that is being labeled carpal tunnel syndrome – and are actually repetitive strain injuries of the various muscles.

As you read the text that is associated with the graphics, you will understand why you don't need carpal tunnel surgery, you only need to release the spasms in the muscles that impact the median nerve! We recommend you click on each link to examine this problem in depth.

To read a clear description of a muscle that raises your arm click on www.aboutcts.com/pectoralis_minor.html. This muscle causes spasms to occur without pain being felt in the area of the spasm, and is a key muscle in the numbness felt in the thumb and fingers.

When a person holds their arm up for extended periods of time, or sleeps with their arm tucked under their head, it may cause hand pain and numbness that is commonly thought of as a symptom of Carpal Tunnel Syndrome. Frequently, because of this reason, people wake up during the night and have to shake out their hand. Releasing the contraction and spasms in the pectoralis minor will return blood flow, and sensation, to the arm and hand. We teach our clients how to change their sleeping habits and keep their arm down during the night.

The median nerve continues to travel under the biceps. One of the branches of the biceps originates on the coracoid process and has the same impact on the median nerve as the pectoralis minor. When the biceps are in contraction they are pulling down on the coracoid process and trapping the nerve under the bone.

It then goes into the forearm where it is frequently trapped by the tight flexor muscles, as shown in http://www.aboutcts.com/flexor_muscles.html.

At the Carpal Tunnel Treatment Center we have found that it is vital to work out each individual spasm in the flexor muscles. Stretching is important, but unless the spasms are released, the muscles cannot be stretched sufficiently to release the strain on the tendons and you develop tendonitis, an inflammation of the tendons.

Most people have heard the term "tendonitis", but they don't realize how a muscle causes this condition.

An analogy we've found useful is to describe the muscle/tendon/bone connection like the system that automatically opens your garage door. The muscle is comparable to the motor of the system, the tendon, a strong fibrous band that connects a muscle to a bone, is like the cable that runs from the motor to the door, and the bone is like the garage door.

When the motor (muscle) is turned on, it pulls on the cable (tendon). The cable then pulls on the door (bone), and the door moves. Likewise, when the muscle pulls on the tendon, the tendon then pulls on the bone and the bone moves.

Look at http://www.aboutcts.com/flexor_muscles.html to view the muscles that enable you to close your hand into a fist and whose tendons pass through the carpal tunnel along with the median nerve.

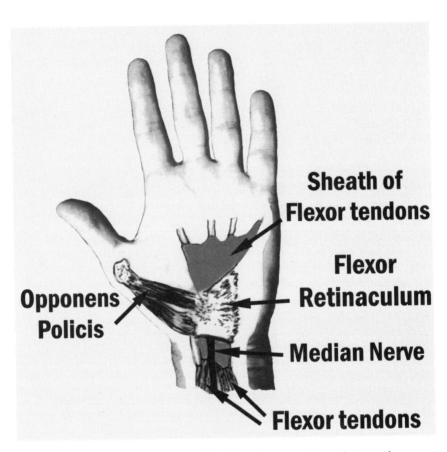

Sheath of Flexor tendons

Flexor Retinaculum

Opponens Policis

Median Nerve

Flexor tendons

The muscle that is responsible for drawing your thumb into the palm of your hand is the opponens pollicis. You can see the muscle, and the bridge by going to:
http://www.aboutcts.com/the_thumb.html.

The thick muscle at the base of the thumb is used millions of times a day. When this muscle is in spasm, it pulls down the roof of the Carpal Tunnel, and puts pressure on the median nerve.

When the flexor muscles, or the thumb muscles, are in spasm they put excessive pressure, or pull, on the carpal tunnel. Often this is tested by an EMG (Electromylogram). An EMG is an unpleasant test frequently used to diagnose Carpal Tunnel Syndrome. An electrode (needle) is placed into a nerve, and a second electrode is placed a distance away. An electrical charge is then passed between the two electrodes.

The technician measures the length of time it takes for the signal to go through the nerve, and if it is delayed you are told you have a "positive" EMG, confirming that you have carpal tunnel syndrome. And you do, but it is because the tendons have trapped the nerve within the tunnel.

At this point you have a few choices. A hand surgeon can cut open the wrist and snip the ligament of the carpal tunnel. However, a much easier approach, and far less painful, is to learn how to treat the spasms of the muscles we have just discussed. This will effectively stop the wrist/hand pain and numbness!

Overuse of anti-inflammatory drugs, and unnecessary surgery, is rampant throughout the USA, causing pain, paralysis, and even death! Dr. Cohen has written an informative pamphlet What You Don't Know CAN Hurt You...7 Important Facts About Carpal Tunnel Syndrome, which you will receive free by going to: http://www.aboutcts.com and registering for the Carpal Tunnel Treatment Center newsletter.

You don't need to open the tunnel – you just need to release the pressure on the nerve!

As mentioned above, Carpal Tunnel Syndrome is the #1 Repetitive Motion Injury in the United States. If you continue doing the movements that are causing the condition, the problem will only get worse.

As you learn how to find and treat the spasms that are pressing on a nerve, you can rest assured that when the repetitive strain injuries of physical activity occur (and they will) anywhere in your body, you will be able to avoid surgery!

CHAPTER 4

Prevent Injuries Through Proper Exercise

By Shawn Boom

It was thirteen hours or so into a mountain biking race that I first noticed the fireflies.

With another twelve hours to go, I took a moment to get off my bike, virtually stopping the race, simply to take in the glowing field of stars on earth.

I was looking down the valley, which I had been biking up and down since noon and thinking how beautiful the 1:00 AM morning was turning out to be. Even through the salted and muddied vision I had earned though the rigors of the race, fireflies somehow became a symbol to me of the great payoffs hard work can lead us to, as athletes, and as people.

In the days preceding the race the butterflies filled my stomach and I was unable to eat. Nervous energy is a challenge for most athletes and it is no different for me. At that point, my last real meal was a few days ago and a combination of physical, emotional and nutritional exhaustion was becoming a near hallucinogenic bliss. Faced with challenges, and motivated by goals, athletes are poised to shine and when they do, the world becomes iridescent in their eyes – it is also this point that the fireflies start to flicker. Like the modern artists of today, this wasn't the first time I've brought myself to tears over the beauty of living life with fireflies as objectives - and it surely wouldn't be the last.

Over the past nine years I've been working hard to become the best person I can be. People choose to pursue the challenge of figuring out who they are in many different ways. So far, my path of self-discovery has taken me through four Ironman Triathlons, one-hundred or so short course triathlons, two 24+ hour cycling races, 19 marathons, a handful of adventure races, world famous rock climbs, volcano and mountain summits and through the ever important college degree (Exercise Physiology, of course). The one thing I have learned through all of these experiences is that the important part of being me is that I am able to share my love for adventure with other people. It is for this reason that I am very pleased to have found Julie Donnelly & Dr. Cohen, and the Julstro techniques. They are dedicated to helping athletes continue to shine by taking both a proactive, and rehabilitation, approach to injured people seeking their own personal fireflies.

I am currently employed by Balanced Body Inc. in the industry of Pilates. I live in Sacramento, California with my wife Bethany, and pug dog Killian. I have coached many people in their first pursuits in sports, and written some fun articles on training. I hope you enjoy the articles and rehab techniques you read in this book, and I welcome any and all comments, criticisms and curiosities.

Everyone has their own firefly; please keep looking for yours.

Shawn Boom

The Physiology of Exercise

Having been an athlete for my entire life, I seem to have acquired a great sense of taste for the adventures and discoveries sports have lent to me. The vagabond nature of my psyche has allowed me to try many different training tactics in pursuit of the highly sought after "fit body". I've done races lasting a matter of seconds..."Dad, I'll race you to the car", up to a matter of days "Hmmm, I guess I can handle sleep deprivation and malnourishment for extended periods of competition".

My point is that I have shaped my life after the pursuit of fitness. My college studies were in Exercise Physiology, I have partaken in endless laboratory experiments that drew blood, measured breathing and calculated power output. I have raced in many Ironman Triathlons, cycled longer than my behind cares to remember, climbed mountains at extreme altitude and fired through adrenaline crushing dares – all to find out how far the human body and mind can be pushed without falling apart.

What I have found by socializing with some of the countries great adventure seekers, and beginner exercises, is that all athletes need to continually learn and think about the inner-workings of their training program if they want to improve their fitness levels and mental attitude, diet, lifestyle factors, and racing seasons.

Many beginners have little concept about the reason they train, other than their personal trainer or coach tells them they really ought to do another set or a few more repetitions. Some long time athletes or "magazine-aholics" out there probably know the variable improvements the human body is capable of making on a biochemical and physiological level. There seems to be an unusual consensus in the fitness industry that knowing what happens to the human body under physical stress and recovery actually assists the body in the process. It is in my opinion that an athlete "doing what they are told" should really be "telling their body what it is going to do". That is to say, getting "in shape" is much easier to do when a person understands what exactly being "in shape" means.

What exactly is "Getting in Shape?"

"Exercise helps you look good naked"... it's a popular slogan many health clubs are using lately, suggesting that if we look good naked we will be "in shape". While changing our physique is often a by-product of exercise, it shouldn't be the prime focus of concern. In general, the human body is capable of reacting to various stimuli as needed.

If a couch potato doesn't offer much in the way of exercise for their body, the body won't offer much in the way of health for said person. If a runner demands that her body perform exercise six to seven days per week, the body will generally respond accordingly. The body's response to what we ask it to do is really where we can find the roots of exercise physiology. Getting in shape is about molding and changing the human body from all levels, beginning with broad changes in things such as our breathing and ending on very specific details like the manipulation of the smallest cellular composition comprehendible to science.

I've got a 'weekend warrior' friend who can model one process by which a hard trying runner gets in shape. Through his racing season, Rusty's body will undergo some very predictable and expected transformations, assuming the training program is put together by someone extremely brilliant and good looking (such as myself). Sometime in the middle of the spring thaw, Rusty knows that he should start training for the summer racing season. Like the good lad that he is, Rusty announces to his friends, "Pals, it's time I began training to increase my capillary functions, improve my ability for rapid fat oxidation, increase my ventilatory capacity, raise my VO2 max, decrease my resting heart rate, raise my lactate threshold, speed my recovery, increase my lean muscle mass, decrease my..." and Rusty's friend cuts him off saying "dude" (yes, Californians still use the word 'dude') you mean you need to get in shape?"

Yes, Rusty is talking about a few of the things that we strive to do when we athletes get in shape. Below you'll notice a list of some things that change inside our bodies when we get "in shape". Think about a typical training week for our weekend warrior runner friend. Aside from the inherent garble of needless responsibilities such as work, laundry, cleaning and family (that is a joke), Rusty is going to give his body somewhere in the neighborhood of five to ten training sessions per week.

Each training session can be quantitatively measured by different things (frequency, intensity, time, sport) and assuming that Rusty's program is laid out correctly, each session will focus on different parts of his physiology, technique and mental toughness. The early parts of the season will be tailored to facilitate physiological adaptation while the middle season training will help him with tuning motor skills and increasing biochemical activities in each little cell. The later portion of Rusty's season will be used to generate muscular power, speed and tapering, respectively.

The major things I encourage athletes to pay attention to in their training are the things that can be measured frequently by themselves that are as non-invasive as possible. Thankfully, exercise labs are not a requisite to becoming a top-notch athlete. While having an exercise physiologist or coach perform specific tests with instruments of elaborate precision is almost always a beneficial learning experience, there are inexpensive tools on the market today that can give you great means by which to assess your current "in-shapeness" as well as serve to be motivating tools.

There are many ways to express exercise intensity:

1. Calories over a given period of time
2. Absolute Power output
3. Perceived Exertion
4. Multiples of resting metabolic rate
5. Relationship of relative metabolic rate relating to Lactate Threshold
6. Relationship of relative metabolic rate relating to VO2 Max
7. Relative percentage of Maximum Heart Rate

Number seven from the above list, Heart Rate, is in my opinion the number one measurement for self coached athlete.

For people new to Heart Rate (Zone) Training, a heart rate monitor comes in two parts. The first part on modern day monitors is a transmitter, generally taking the form of a chest strap. The second part of the equation is a wristwatch that gathers electrical impulses sent from the transmitter and relates them into information called "Beats Per Minute (BPM)". This number is the amount of beats an athletes heart is beating per minute and in my estimation training with this number in mind is one of the single most accurate ways to get in shape. If you are an athlete without a heart rate monitor find a way to gain access to one – they are extremely economical today.

When am I officially in shape?

I hear this question all of the time. Generally it is presented to me in the form of a statement such as, "I need to lose ten pounds" with the inference being that the 10 extra pounds is really what is keeping that person from being in shape. Incidentally enough, the loss of those ten pounds (as described above) is simply a by-product of other changes occurring within the body. The starting point for beginner and elite athletes who want to perform to the best of their physiological abilities is to regularly document their workout measurements in a training log. There are a good number of computer software programs on the market for the tech-geeks, and there are double the amounts of great workout logbooks for sale in print. I simply use a plain printed calendar with a month and week view. Whatever your choice, arm yourself first with this calendar and an accompanying 3-ring binder folder. The binder will be used to collect articles, document test results, write down notes and tips, and collect whatever other useful tidbits you find. Remember, sports are just as much about the educational side of the game as they are the physical.

The human mind has proven over and again its capabilities to directly influence racing performance, training results and yes, aesthetic appearances (for you who haven't quite caught on to the whole point of this article yet). The real answer to the question "When am I officially in shape?" is that regardless of your current starting point, once you show that you are on a linear line of continual improvements, you are getting in shape! This line isn't just a theoretical; it is a positive line you can document in measurable terms.

General Fitness Assessment Tests

The first thing you need to do is assess your current physical condition. If you haven't worked out in the past 12 months, do yourself a favor and swallow your pride by visiting a doctor. Assuming you are healthy and ready to begin a training program (or begin training at a higher level, for you elites), you will need to learn your maximum heart rate. There are many ways to access tests offering this information. One of the greatest resources I can lend you to is my friend Sally Edwards. After finishing 16 Ironman Triathlons, Sally was inducted into the Triathlon Hall of Fame! Please take a few moments now and visit her website at http://www.Heartzones.com. While you are there, choose a protocol for calculating your max heart rate and get outside to take the test. Once you have that number written down in your 3-ring binder, revisit the tests below. If you don't currently have a heart rate monitor, please beg, borrow or steal one because a serious athlete cannot move forward without knowing their five heart rate zones. If you have any questions, contact staff@heartzone.com.

Armed with your max heart rate numbers, the next tests I will encourage you to take include:

- The Anaerobic Threshold
- The one-mile running heart rate test
- The 10 mile cycling heart rate test
- The recovery heart rate test

At the very least, you should build each of these tests into your training regime once each month. By continually monitoring the results (and ideally graphing them out in a computer spreadsheet program) you will become familiar with many of the changes your body is making while you train. When you have test results for the above five test, I'd say you're in pretty good shape already!

Remembering here that the goal of training is to develop stronger muscles, a healthier heart, better functioning joints, and an overall feeling of euphoria for life, spend some time listening to your body and how it reacts to the exercise you have given it today. Your body will, in turn, react to you in the way that you ask of it.

CHAPTER 5

The Core Workouts of Fast Triathletes – Part I

Shawn Boom

When I want to climb a mountain, I train by hiking, climbing and running and weight lifting the certain muscles I know I'm going to need during my big day. When I want to hit a baseball really far, I spend time working on my technique of swinging a bat and weight training specific muscle movements I know I'll need during the big game.

Likewise, when I want to compete fast (or just simply finish a race for that matter) I follow the principle of exercise called "sport specific training". This means that not only do I run and weight lift but I do them in a systematic and scientific approach so that on race day I can show up with confidence and a finely tuned body.

Sports specific training in means that the exercises and workout sessions an athlete does won't be of much benefit to the race unless it is either building strength for muscles or joints, helping with movement pattern training or conditioning the same metabolic pathways that will be used during the race itself. Keeping this principle in mind, the following is an infrastructure of a training program I use when training athletes I am coaching — as well as myself.

The Principle of Three

There are three essential workouts that occur in a regular training week for every advanced runner. Being that there are only a limited number of hours in a day, and unless you can take time off work, which I encourage if possible, many athletes hit the wall of life everyday. There comes a point, just like in races, that reality becomes the strongest beast inside the body and we can't go on with training unlimited amounts of time. When the garden hedges need cutting, the garage needs cleaning and the weekend is almost over, we all realize that there needs to be a concise and spelled out formula for getting and staying in shape. The three key workouts have been suggested by many before me and will be used by many after me. Nonetheless, utilizing these key workouts each week is a great goal to begin with.

THREE KEY WEEKLY WORKOUTS

Intervals

An interval is a repeat of low (easy effort) and high (hard effort) stress that results in the body's adaptation to a new and higher level of fitness. Interval training is a methodology of training that includes regular doses of low and high repeats of training.

Threshold workout

This workout is your favorite activity performed at moderate intensity. For me, it's a certain run I do down the river trail, or my morning bike ride that can be done easily before work. These workouts are moderate intensity, normally Zone 3 (70-80% MHR), and last about as long as the interval workouts ... but they're much easier.

Long workout

A long workout should be performed each week at a low intensity. For your long workouts, begin by doing one each week for 7 weeks. However long the long workout is, it should be based on time, not distance. Go at 70% for 7 weeks during this workout.

Take a look at your workout week. If you can't find each of these three types of workouts, tweak one of them to become one of these! Each of these workouts stresses your body a bit differently, teaching your cells and muscles to utilize different metabolic pathways, and helping you reach your goal in a systematic and effective manner.

The three-workout rule suggests that each week a triathlete will complete an "Interval", "Threshold" and "Long" workout.

This concept is based on the principles of adaptation and progression. As you become more fit, you can train at higher intensities and for longer periods of time using lower amounts of energy. By stressing the body in different ways, you are able to build a highly trained system of biological pathways that accommodate hard training efforts with the necessary physiological components as well as aid in healing when you train at lower levels.

Plateau

These workouts (long workout, threshold and interval workout) are all that is needed to help an athlete attain and maintain a certain level of fitness. Anything above and beyond these workouts is not necessary, though not necessarily harmful. A great runner can win races on this formula and a beginner will finish with incredible confidence by working her way up to this level. As progression and adaptation occur, athletes need to continue to change their training pattern (by varying there phases as discussed below and by including cross-training and weight lifting).

We can further break a training season down into four phases: Base, Speed, Power, and Peak. Depending on what point in the training season an athlete is, the time and intensity of these workouts will vary greatly.

A reasonable training cycle for a beginning triathlete would allow for 4 – 6 weeks of base training, 3 weeks of speed training, little or no time spent in power training and about 1 week spent "peaking". See the sidebar for more details on this terminology. This means that a beginner would need to start training no less than 8 weeks prior to their first race. I also don't recommend that beginners jump into a race that exceeds their longest training workout by 2 times. This means that if the longest workout a new triathlete has finished is one hour, then a race lasting longer than 2 hours should be reconsidered.

Four Phases of Training

While training theories differ throughout the world, the reoccurring theme infers that cycling the training doses is the most effective way to condition one's body to perform at a high level. Keeping in mind that "high level" is a relative term and that finishing a race might be a high level to one person and a simple expectation to another. The following are four general categories of training cycles I use when putting together all athletes training programs. The time allotted to each phase of training is a general statement and is transient based on past training experience. In addition, the following recommendations are based on portions of my personal experience as a triathlon coach and athlete, and represent my training philosophy, which has been shaped by a great number of teachers and researchers.

Base Training

2-8 weeks: Training done for longer periods of time at lower intensities. If measuring with a heart rate monitor, it is recommended that those in the base training phase train no higher than 70% of their max heart rate. Base training helps with anatomical adaptation including the strengthening of tendons and ligaments, increasing the red blood cell count, helping the body appropriately burn the correct combination of fats and carbohydrates, and much more.

Speed Training

2-4 weeks: After the base building phase, an athlete is generally overtaken with boredom and a strong desire to "go faster". Because 70% of max heart rate (MHR) is usually a slow pace for most athletes, speed training comes as a great relief and a welcome change. The first few weeks of speed training should concentrate on building strength more than speed. I generally like to spend 2 weeks doing ? of the amount of intervals I plan on accomplishing at the end of the speed session. For example, if I'm allowing my body 4 weeks of speed training by which at the end I plan on running 6 x 1 mile repeats at 85% MHR, I will spend the first two weeks building up from 3 or 4 miles at 80-85% MHR followed by some sports specific weight lifting (with repetitions of about 12-15).

I allow my body adequate base building and strength adaptation periods because I know my muscles are capable of getting stronger a lot faster than my tendons and ligaments. After a few weeks of light speed/strength training, my muscles are probably adapting and growing but my joints will lag behind a little bit. By slowing growing into the speed training, I am certain that I won't be hurt when it comes time to train hard. There is a tendency to go faster than necessary at an early point in the season and it can be detrimental to your training and life if you don't follow the principles of adaptation and progression. When beginning the speed-training phase, always pay close attention to the small changes and warning signals your body gives. If you feel a new "twinge" or a muscle that just "doesn't feel right", take a day or two completely off – because a few days of self treatment beats a few months of inactive living on the couch!

Power Training

2-3 weeks: Beginning triathletes will want to avoid this training phase of 3 weeks if they don't have previous experience with high intensity training. Advanced triathletes can use this phase for no more than three weeks without planning a new recovery cycle. The power workouts can do incredible harm to the muscular anatomy of a person who isn't well adapted. For this reason, I recommend that anyone planning to enter the power phase of training cycle through 2 speed phases (3 weeks each with one week recovery between) in order to adapt and progress to a point where injury can hopefully be avoided and at worst be limited. Power workouts for runners include moderate time investments with maximum power output.

Running on hills, cycling on a wind-trainer so as not to be interrupted by traffic, swimming high volume intervals and lifting more weights with less reps are included in the power training phase. Efforts last anywhere from 3 minutes in the pool to 10 minutes on the bike to 6 minutes running. Heart rates will exceed 93-95% MHR and adequate dietary intake is a must. If a beginner athlete wishes to skip the power phase, they can either choose to recycle through another speed phase (not changing intensity but adding time) or altogether advance to the peaking phase.

In the power phase, the adaptation and progression concept plays out in an obvious manner. By progressively lowering the number of reps or intervals and raising the intensity level or weights, the body is forced to do greater amounts of work output. Providing that there is a substantial recovery period between each hill, repeat or lift, the body will be capable of performing repeated exercises at highly intense levels. It is important to remember the principles of the nine-workout rule – just because this is the power phase doesn't mean that every workout is done as a power workout. The concepts of nine key workouts still applies, this phase just means that when intervals are part of a workout, they are done as outlined by the principles of power training. It is also important to note that the body doesn't get stronger while performing exercise; it actually breaks down while training.

The building up of our muscles and cells occurs in the times of our lives when we are recovering, such as sitting at our desk in the office, sleeping and stretching. When training at high levels, be sure to give intense rest periods to your body as well. Think of rest like a supplemental vitamin that aids in recovery. It is especially important to self-administer precautionary treatments to the body's muscles and cells. Eating good food is always important but having the correct balance when training in the power phase is highly related to muscle and joint recovery. Massage is always a good tool of injury prevention, as are proactive thermal treatments of contrasting temperatures.

Peaking

1 - 2 weeks: The peak training phase is where you can fine-tune your body and your equipment. About 2 1/2 weeks before the major race of the season, take in your last long workout. In the middle of the long workout, if you feel inspired, throw in some moderate intervals that slowly raise your heart rate by 10% of your race pace, lasting from 10 to 15 minutes. In the two weeks immediately after your last long workout, cut your workout time down to 45 minutes for beginners and no more than 1 hour and 15 minutes for Marathon Runners. During these last workouts, take a lot of recovery time and low heart rate training with the intermixing of some speed training, equivalent in intensity but less time that where you ended in the last speed phase of your training. This is the time when you should feel light on your feet, anxious and full of energy.

A well peaked athlete often gets crabby because the volume of training they are used to is cut back up to 50% and the usual energy outlet that once existed is no longer a viable option. There will be more time available in a runners day when she is peaking and I recommend doing light stretching and spending extra down time partaking in mind-body exercises.

Don't do anything "new" for exercise in the peaking phase. Plan to be "in shape" for yoga, Pilates, or whatever other supplemental training regimes you plan to use while peaking. I had a friend injure himself during the final training sessions prior to a big race simply because with a decrease in training volume he got bored and started playing softball for fun. The last time he had swung a bat was in high school and his triathlon was a miserable experience because he got to know the meaning of back spasms! During the Peaking phase, spend time concentrating on the race and enjoying time with your family – don't try anything new!

A Closer Look at the Key Weekly Workouts

The Long Workout

The purpose of the long workout each week is to develop and maintain a "base" as it is commonly referred to. Having a base is almost as elusive as being "in shape". There is no checkpoint by which one can determine they either have or have not established a base. Using the continuous measurement system outline in the above tests, one can, however, determine the movements of their physiological patterns and be able to study their own body's reaction to training doses.

In addition to working on an athlete's base, a long workout provides the joints and bones an opportunity to get used to working for a long time and offers the adequate time for building a stronger infrastructure.

The Threshold Workout

Of the many thresholds in an athlete's life, there are two very important ones to consider in the threshold workout. The first is called the aerobic threshold and generally falls between 50-55% of one's maximum heart rate. Workouts below this intensity are not really considered to be "workouts". That said, there are numerous benefits to training inside the aerobic workout, such as increased ability for tendons and ligaments to adapt to exercise before stressing them in harder workouts. Other benefits arise in the form fuel usage. It is in the aerobic threshold workouts that a person burns the highest percentage of fat as a fuel source.

Because through a complex series of chemical reactions, fat needs oxygen present (80-85% of the total calories burned here are fat calories).

The Interval Workout

By introducing interval training into a weekly workout regime, athletes become aware of many benefits not fully realized by regular training. While all athletes can derive benefit from interval training, I recommend that only experienced athletes partake in any intervals that take their heart rate over 90% of maximum. Intervals mean that training intensities vary in incremental units based on time, distance or a combination thereof. Common ways to denote intervals in a training program (and the way I use in this book) are as follows:

What the Workout Says	What the workout Means
4 x 1 mile @ 87% MHR on with 1.5 times rest	4 intervals of 1 mile each. Each interval is done at an effort of 807% of one's individual max heart rate. Whatever time the athlete finished the miles should be multiplied by 1.5 to determine rest time
8 x 1000 meters @ 90% MHR with 3 minutes recovery or to 65% MHR	8 intervals of 1000 meters each, performed at 90 percent of one's maximum heart rate. Time is not the determining factor in this kind of workout ~ recovery (measured by heart rate) is the indicator flag to watch. When an athlete finishes one of these intervals, they are free to begin the next immediately when their heart rate recovers to 65% of maximum heart rate.

Example: Running Interval Workout

	Intervals	Endurance	Anaerobic Threshold
Example Workout	4 x 1 mile @ 87%+ MHR with equal or 1.5 times recovery	8-15+ miles @ 60-70% MHR depending on distance of last long run	8 x 1000 meters at 90% MHR with 3 minutes recovery
Training Benefit	Increased recovery, higher tolerance to lactic acid, increased VO2 Max	Anatomical Adaptation	Increase in Anaerobic Threshold, increased anaerobic enzymes for more efficient use of fat as a fuel source at higher intensities, heart rate efficiency

Intervals like the example above are great because they allow for greater efforts over a shorter period of time. Don't be fooled, however – intervals can be done lower levels of intensity too – and in any sports that you cross train in (swimming, cycling, inline skating, etc.)

The Core Workouts of Fast Triathletes – Part II

Shawn Boom

The following workouts are what I consider to be the best application of speed and stress upon a long distance triathlete's body. The theories behind them, however, are very applicable to any triathlete training for any distance. They are written specifically for long course racers (i.e. Half-Ironman and Ironman distances).

Common Triathlon Distances

Sprint
There is no standard sprint distance. Anything less than Olympic Distance is considered a sprint.

Olympic (International):
1.5K swim, 40K bike, 10K run

Half-Ironman:
1.2-mile swim, 56-mile bike, 13.1 mile run

Ironman:
2.4-mile swim, 112-mile bike, 26.2 mile run

Short course Triathletes will need to modify the distances to an appropriate ratio for their intended race length. It would suffice to say that an Olympic Distance racing doesn't require more than a 3 hour bike ride or 2 hour run at anytime during the training or racing season and that any workouts exceeding these time limits should be cut back by time, not distance, to fall within the ranges given in the chart to the right. The purpose of stressing the body is to recover adequately afterward.

It is essential that when you complete the following workouts, you maintain the proper stretching, diet, and sleep patterns. The time you are resting is the time that your muscles need to build and repair themselves. These workouts are hard, demand you to be rested when completing them, and WILL WORK if you punch out the effort they require. They are for high performance Triathletes, have been created by me over years of elite racing experience, and are here to make you fast.

Before offering sample workouts, it is important to note that any training done on questionable injuries is not recommended under any circumstance. It is far better to lose two weeks of training than to put forth an effort to continue working out on injuries and risk missing an entire season. When injuries occur, and they will, follow the recommended treatment protocols in this book before continuing on.

Recommended Training Accomplishments

Training distances vary greatly from one triathlete to the next. The amount of time one-person trains for a sprint distance triathlon might very well be enough to get them through an Olympic distance race. Likewise, a person gearing up for an Ironman might be doing the same training plan someone getting ready for half that distance is using. The following are recommended ranges of training time spent per session. They are goal times, giving a range of the minimum and maximum training levels necessary for a person to feel comfortable finishing their given race distance. For example, if you are training for an Olympic Distance triathlon, you should at least be able to swim for 30 minutes, bike for 1.5 hours and run for an hour – however it wouldn't be necessary to have swam over one hour, biked more than three or run past 2 hours. The important point it to take note of the maximum time necessary for each discipline. This chart does not give mention to intensity because these are training times necessary for one to simply complete a race. It is inferred that training intensities will be cycled accordingly and that the triathlete will race in direct proportion to how well trained they are.

	SWIMMING		BIKING		RUNNING	
	MINIMUM ACCEPTABLE	MAXIMUM NECESSARY	MINIMUM ACCEPTABLE	MAXIMUM NECESSARY	MINIMUM ACCEPTABLE	MAXIMUM NECESSARY
Sprint	20 min.	30 min.	45 min.	1 hour	20 min.	45 min.
Olympic	30 min.	1 hours	1.5 hours	3 hours	1 hour	2 hours
Half Ironman	40 min.	1 hour 20 min.	3 hours	4 hours	2 hours	3 hours
Ironman+	1 hour	2 hours	5 hours	7 hours	2.5 hr	4 hours

Functions of Training for Triathlon Swimming

The strategy for triathlon swimming is much different than swimming only competitions. A triathlete must use her legs later in the race, and therefore preserve the glycogen (simple sugar) stores so for cycling and running. Because of this it is important that a triathlete train using a 2 or 4 beat kick rather than the traditional infinite fluttering a sprint swimmer uses. For details on how to train your swimming

Reading a Swim workout

*   5 x 100 is read five by one-hundred and means you swim 100 meters 5 times.

•   5 x 100 on 2:00 is read five by one-hundred on two minutes and means that on every two-minute mark, you begin your next interval. (i.e. the faster you swim, the longer your rest).

•   SKPS means swim, kick, pull, swim. It is a good way to warm up, cool down, break up hard interval sets and relieve boredom.

technique for triathlons, I recommend checking out http://www.TotalImmersion.com

My swimming programs follow the 9 key workout principle. The three key workouts that swimming adds to the total are:

1.   Intervals

2.   Drills

3.   Long Swims

For swimmers and Triathletes with a solid background in the pool, there is not as much of a need to train for swimming fitness until the 8 weeks prior to a race. Having finished 3 Ironman Triathlon and a hundred or so Olympic distances, I have run the gamut of swimming session per week from minimum to maximum. At one point, I was in the pool 6 days a week for 10 months training for an Ironman. The next Ironman I did, I swam 2 times per week for 4 weeks before the race. Albeit, the second Ironman was a bit more painful, my time was only thirty-seconds slower than the first. I have since decided upon a compromise and I now begin my swim training 8 weeks prior to the race, three sessions per week for using the above three workouts per week. My background is strong in swimming, however. If you are like most Triathletes, you'll want to make more of a buildup to race day. In this case, double up on the drills workout.

Beginner swimmers will range from never having put their face in the water to lifetime fish in need of some simple technique work. I recommend that when starting a swimming program, most of the beginning month be comprised mainly of technique and stroke drills. Not only are they tiring but they will give you more bang for your buck when it comes to race day. If you are relatively new to this triathlon gig, enlist in your local masters swimming program and put in some time doing laps with other people.

Only you know where your comfort level is in the water. Keeping in mind that triathlons are about breaking outside of your comfort levels, be fair with yourself in your estimation of your swimming abilities. The following workouts provide 3 weeks worth of examples of key swimming workouts I use when training elite swimmers – and I've made variations to accommodate beginners as well. Have fun in designing your swims and remember triathlons have no rules about what strokes you use, so do whatever is comfortable for you.

Any of the following workouts can be modified for various distances. It is also important to note that these workouts are not written in a progression based model, meaning that they are examples of workouts from various weeks during the training season and don't represent the first three weeks in a row of training. The purpose of these workouts are to give you an overview of some types of workouts both advanced and beginners alike can modify to fit their talents, goals, and needs. For a tailored training plan for you, please email shawn@cwnet.com.

Note: All distances listed below are in meters.

Week #1 Swimming Workouts

1. Intervals

200 SKPS:	800
200 Pull:	200
5x50 Swim on 1 min	250
5x100 Swim on 2 min	500
200 Cool Down	<u>200</u>
	1950

2. Drills

100 SKPS	400
All Drills x 50	600
500 Swim	<u>500</u>
	1500

3. Long Swim

Open Water: 40-50 Min or extended long swim in the pools with open water technique. Go for time, not yardage.

Week #2 Swimming Workouts

1. Intervals

400 Warm-up	400
5x250 on 6:00	1,250
3x25 sprint on 1:00	75
75 cool down- Arms don't come out of the water.	75
	1,800

2. Drills

150 SPS	450
Pulling Drills x 50	200
Catch Up	
One Arm (each arm)	
Finger Tip Drag	
Monkey Swim	
10 x 50 (25 drill, 25 swim)	500
Take as long as you need. You choose the drills.	1150

3. Long Swim

Open Water:	Minutes
5:00 easy, 5:00 hard	10:00
4:00 easy, 4:00 hard	8:00
3:00 easy, 3:00 hard	6:00
2:00 easy, 2:00 hard	4:00
1:00 easy, 1:00 hard	2:00
Cool-down 10:00 -	12:00
hands may not leave the water.	40:00

This workout may be substituted with the pool version called, "5 and Down" in the key swim workout pages

Week #3 Swimming Workouts

1. Intervals

250 SKPS	1,000
3 x 500 on 9 min. –	
Long rest periods so go hard.	1,500
500 drills	<u>500</u>
	2,000

2. Drills

"Only Drills Day"	
100 warm up	100
4 x 50, each drill	<u>1,200</u>
	1,300

3. Long Swim

100 SKPS	400
2 x 1000 at race pace	2,000
3 x 200 focus on technique	<u>600</u>
	3,000

Swim Key Workouts

The above workouts are examples of how a swimming program is laid out. After an initiation period with an athlete (or with yourself if you are a self-coached athlete) these workouts would be adjusted appropriately according to your race distance, training limitations and goals. Using workouts such as these, you will build up to higher intensities, lower rest, and longer distances. The key thing to remember, as outlined above, is that there are always three key workouts to complete for each discipline. For swimming, those workouts are: Intervals, Drills and Long Swims.

In addition to the requisite three training sessions each week, I like to add in what I consider to be "key workouts". They are the centerpoint of my training cycles and every time I want to test my fitness I use them as a base by which to compare my improvements. The principle factor to remember when creating or completing key workouts for yourself is that they should always limit variabilities as much as possible. For instance, in swimming I always pick a nice still day with no wind, good temperate, and adequate rest prior to the workout. I want to start the key workouts feeling rested, almost like a "mini-taper" before the test.

In swimming, I use two workouts and try to monitor my two-minute recovery heart rate at the end of the intervals and workout itself. Anyone ever having tried to keep the heart transmitter on their chest during a swim workout knows this isn't an easy task. Women have a simple solution, which is to purchase a swimsuit that accommodates a heart monitor transmitter by offering a slot in the material itself. Men have a simple solution to – duct tape. I'm not kidding, shave your chest and tape that transmitter to you – it's either tape or a woman's swimsuit, your choice. If none of the above solutions are acceptable to you, I can't say I blame you. For the less hard-core of us, simply leaving the transmitter at pool edge will suffice as you can easily hold it up to your chest upon completion of each interval. Still, it is felt by many that duct tape proves your dedication though. Oh, and I'm not liable for this suggestion.

Feel free to invent your own key workouts, the following are two that I enjoy as a test and also as a way to keep myself on track and having a good time.

Swim Key Workout #1 – "5 And Down"

This workout is best used for one of two reasons. First, if you haven't been swimming much but are in fair swim shape, it brings you back up to speed fast. Second, if you are preparing for a long race, this workout is an excellent race prep workout because it allows you to burst out of your speed for a time and teaches recovery while swimming (such is the technique a triathlete would use to flow from pack to pack in the race). It is a great pool workout and relieves much of the monotony. An eager open water swimmer can use this workout by going by time, not distance. A beginning swimmer or short course triathlete will find benefit in completing the same distances below with a higher intensity of "on" or "hard" intervals and a slower and lazier recovery "off" or "easy" intervals.

5 and Down – by distance	
500 easy, 500 hard	1,000
400 easy, 400 hard	800
300 easy, 300 hard	600
200 easy, 200 hard	400
100 easy, 100 hard	200
100 cool-down with arms NOT leaving the water	<u>100</u>
	3,100

5 and Down – by time	
Open Water:	*Minutes*
5:00 easy, 5:00 hard	10:00
4:00 easy, 4:00 hard	8:00
3:00 easy, 3:00 hard	6:00
2:00 easy, 2:00 hard	4:00
1:00 easy, 1:00 hard	2:00
10:00 cool-down; hands may not leave the water.	<u>12:00</u>
	40:00

Swim Key Workout #2 – Ironman Prep Swim

This workout is a long swim. The best way to use this workout is to do it 5 times from the week that lies 7 weeks from race day through the week that lies 2 weeks from race day. (I.e. if the race is June 1st, then at about April 6th – May 18th would be the period of time for it). The goal here is efficient use of non-biking and running muscles and extending the endurance in your stroke. If you are doing a half Ironman, you may cut the 1000's down to 2 instead of 4, making the workout 4,100 meters! Olympic Distance racers and beginners may cut down the SKPS's to 250 meters and the 1000's to 2 sets, making the workout 3,100 meters!

500 SKPS	2,000
4 x 1000 swim with 5 minutes recovery	4,000
100 cool down	100
	6,100

Functions of Training for Triathlon Cycling

Cycling in triathlons is extremely different than cycling as a sport itself. Many people feel that a triathlon is won or lost on the bike. Beginners tend to like cycling the most, probably because it is a non-impact exercise that doesn't require the support of one's entire body weight. While an elite biker would probably disagree with the idea that cycling is the easiest of the three-triathlon disciplines, it is always a great way for Triathletes to enjoy great fitness benefits and performance improvements.

I won't get too detailed on the technical side of cycling. Suffice it to say that many things on a triathlete's bike are very different from other modalities of biking. ANY bike will work for a triathlon; however, Elite racers will find that strict competition rules dictate makeups of their bike ranging from varying angles to weight limits. Beginner and intermediate triathletes need not worry about such rules; nobody can take away your inner feelings of accomplishment for even starting a race, much less finishing it using the greatest gear or newest accessories.

The following are example workouts for three weeks. Again, these workouts reiterate the 9 key workout principle, providing three major cycling workouts per week in the following three categories of training:

1. Intervals

2. Long Workout

3. Threshold Workout

Any of the following workouts can be modified for various distances. In general, they are written for Olympic or Half Ironman triathletes and will need to be lengthened for Ironman triathletes and shortened for Sprint triathlete and beginner Olympic Distance racers. Always remember to go at your own pace and distance, and keep it fun.

Any of the following workouts can be modified for various distances. It is also important to note that these workouts are not written in a progression based model, meaning that they are example workouts from various weeks during the training season and don't represent the first three weeks in a row of training. The purpose of these workouts are to give you an overview of some types of workouts both advanced and beginners alike can modify to fit their talents, goals, and needs. For a tailored training plan for you, please email shawn@cwnet.com.

Week #1 Cycling Workouts

Intervals

15 Min warm-up @ 70% Maximum Heart Rate

5 x 3 miles as close to 90% MHR as you can hold.

Pedal 1 mile very easy for recovery between each interval

Cool down for 10-15 minutes.

Threshold Workout

10-15 minute warm up at 70% MHR

Go to 75% MHR and hold steady for 5 minutes

Go to 80% MHR and hold steady for 4 minutes

Go to 85% MHR and hold steady for 3 minutes

Go to 90% MHR and hold steady for 2 minutes

Go to 85% MHR and hold steady for 3 minutes

Go to 80% MHR and hold steady for 4 minutes

Go to 75% MHR and hold steady for 5 minutes

Repeat if long course triathlete, or double the times spent at each interval.

10 minute cool down.

Long Ride

1 hr 50 min as follows:

20 min extended warm up @ 70%

30 min @80%

1 hr. @ 85%

If it's too hard to hold the last hour @ 85%, cross up and down from 70-85% every 5 minutes.

Week #2 Cycling Workouts

Intervals

Note: Do this workout in the Power phase of training.

Hills: Find a hill you can punch up in a very low (hard) gear and still stay on your aero bars. If you can't find a hill, do the time on your trainer and elevate the front tire to knee level. Push through the pedal stroke with your heal leading. Do this workout on the hill and work on POWER.

> 10 x 2 minutes @ 80-90% with 45 sec. Rest between.

Threshold Workout

> 10 minutes warm up @ 70% MHR
>
> 3 x 20 minutes at 5 beats above race pace
>
> *Rest 5 minutes between intervals
>
> Cool Down 10-15 minutes at 70% or less

Long Ride

> 2 1/2 –3 hours @ 10 beats below Anaerobic Threshold from Tuesday.

This workout is to test race pace. Notice how you feel during the ride and assess the intensity level as if it were preceding a run.

Week #3 Cycling Workouts

Intervals

Warm Up

Light bike @70%. Do bursts up to 90% every 5 minutes and once you get there, 5 beats every 45 seconds until you get back down to 70%. Use high (easy) gearing.

Threshold Workout

Warm Up for 15 minutes

4 x 5 miles @ Anaerobic Threshold Heart Rate (if you don't know it, take the Anaerobic Threshold test for cycling)

*Rest 1 mile at 60-70% Maximum Heart Rate.

Long Ride

3/4th of your race distance @ 5 beats below race pace. Ideally, this ride would be followed by a race pace run the next day lasting for 30 minutes to one hour, depending on the length of the race (shorter races would be closer to 30 minutes, longer races closer to one-hour).

Bike Key Workouts

Bike Key Workout #1 – Raise Your Anaerobic Threshold

Anaerobic threshold is the point where you are using less oxygen that your muscles need for fat metabolism. It is most accurately assessed in an exercise laboratory but can be done on your own with a heart rate monitor. Since above anaerobic threshold, muscles are using less fat and more carbohydrate, our muscles are left with less net energy to use- because we hold unlimited amounts of fat in our bodies, but the carbohydrate stores are mainly limited by the amount of glycogen in our blood. AT is a transient number- it CAN move up or down, as you get more or less fit. As you get more fit, your AT moves up; so the goal is to raise "AT". When AT is raised, fat can be burned as a fuel source at higher levels of intensity. The only way to raise the anaerobic threshold it to train above it! This interval workout is a great way to raise your anaerobic threshold closer to your max heart rate. Keeping in mind that most people's anaerobic threshold lies between 80 and 90% MHR, elite athletes nearly always hold theirs in the 90-95% MHR range; the higher, the better, as it ultimately tells you how fast you can race without "bonking". You have to know your cycling AT before doing this workout.

> 15 minutes warm up @ 70% MHR
>
> 5 to 10 x 2.5 miles @ 5-8 beats higher than your current AT
>
> 10 minute cool-down @ 70% MHR.

Bike Key Workout #2 – Anaerobic Threshold Test

Providing you have adequate amounts of rest, along side neutral weather conditions, this workout is one of the best to monitor your training progression. I personally use this every two weeks in place of my threshold workout.

> Warm up
>
> 2 x 20 minutes as hard as you can go (active rest between intervals)
>
> Cool down

Bike Key Workout #3 – Lactic Threshold Workout

This workout is to raise your tolerance to the poison, lactic acid, which your body produces when you "go hard". The only way to make your muscles function effectively in the presence of this toxin is to train them to "ignore" it as much as possible. You have to do this hard to make it work- and I suggest you do it on an indoor trainer if you don't have access to a long flat stretch of road that doesn't make you stop for cars, stop signs, or other obstacles that throw off your timing. Beginning Triathletes should do this workout without the 10-second sprints, as their goal in the race is to finish, which doesn't require doing the race over lactic threshold anyway.

---

20 minute warm up

4 x 5 minutes @ 85% MHR. Recover 2 ? minutes between intervals with an easy pedal at 60% MHR.

20 minutes: every minute, on the minute, get up and sprint for 10 seconds.

15 minutes @ 70% for cool-down.

Functions of Training for Triathlon Running

Triathlon running is a tough method to learn. Even very quick athletes with solid distance running backgrounds are dumbfounded initially by the adjustment required to run after swimming and cycling. Beginner triathletes who are intimidated by the idea of even participating in a triathlon are often times put at ease with the idea that the "run" can actually be a "walk", both in training AND in racing. There is no rule that says a triathlete has to run the race and most certainly anyone wanting to merely finish the race, which is a victory in itself, can always hold tight to this security blanket.

Walking is a form of running many elite triathletes become aware of too, most often after a day of hard racing when proper training or nutrition was for one reason or another not part of their race mix. A very high percentage of Ironman triathletes end up walking in their races. There is no shame in finishing, but everyone will admit that it is a little more fun (and sometimes gratifying to the ego) when you can finish with flair.

The following are example workouts for three weeks of triathlon running. Again, these workouts reiterate the 9 key workout principle, providing three major cycling workouts per week in the following three categories of training:

- Intervals

- Long Workout

- Threshold Workout

Any of the following workouts can be modified for various distances. It is also important to note that these workouts are not written in a progression based model, meaning that they are example workouts from various weeks during the training season and don't represent the first three weeks in a row of training. The purpose of these workouts are to give you an overview of some types of workouts both advanced and beginners alike can modify to fit their talents, goals, and needs. For a tailored training plan for you, please email shawn@cwnet.com.

Week #1 Running Workouts

Intervals

> Warm Up
>
> Short course triathletes: 12 x 400 meters @ 90-93% MHR
>
> Long course triathletes: 5 x 6 minutes at 87-90% MHR
>
> Cool Down

Threshold Workout

"Anaerobic Threshold Test"

> Warm Up to your comfort level
>
> 2 x 20 minutes as hard as you can go (active rest between intervals)
>
> Cool down

The average of your heart rates for the first 20 minutes and the second 20 minutes, averaged together is your approximate anaerobic threshold heart rate. For example, if I averaged 180 beats in the first 20 minutes and 190 beats in the second, my estimated anaerobic threshold heart rate would be

(180 + 190) / 2 = 185

Long Run

1 hr. 15 min @ 75-85% MHR. The goal here being to maintain a steady heart rate throughout the entire long run. Experienced athletes and beginners alike should stick to the time provided and put their mental efforts into holding as steady a heart rate as possible.

Week #2 Running Workouts

Intervals

Note: Do this workout in the Power phase of training.

---

6 x 2 minute hills

Find a hill that takes about 2 minutes. Run up it at 87% and recover back down to 60%. Repeat 6 times. Warm up and cool down 15 minutes each.

Threshold Workout

---

20 minute warm up.

4 x 5 minutes at your anaerobic threshold +3 beats

Cool down 25 min.

Long Run

---

2 hr 30 minutes @ 5-8 Beats below AT running AT

Test your race pace of 5—8 beats lower than AT for long course. Short course triathletes should cut the time down to 2 hours and concentrate on their race pace being around (or above AT) which means the long run shouldn't be run at race pace.

Week #3 Running Workouts

Intervals

20 Min warm up

15 min @ 88%

8 min @ 64%

10 min @ 89%

8 min @ 63 %

5 min @ 90%

Cool down 5 min @ 60 %

Threshold Workout

9 Miles (beginners, cut this distance to 6 miles total)

Warm Up 20 min.

Do 8 x 5 minutes @AT +3.

Recover 3 minutes at 60% between intervals.

Focus on building strength and endurance in the intervals.

Cool Down 10 + min

Long Run

3 hours @ AT pace minus 5 beats. Test this pace and heart rate and see how it feels. If you are unable to sustain the pace, drop another 5 beats. Decide what heart rate you want to race your triathlon at. Olympic distance triathletes should cut this workout to 2 hours in length and aim for a pace of AT minus 3 beats.

Running Key Workouts

Run Key Workout #1 - 20, 15, 10, 5 Run Workout

The greatest way to improve your endurance is doing interval workouts that make you recover at a high percentage of your max heart rate. This one should be done anytime during your periodization cycle after your base phase is complete. You have to know your AT before doing this workout.

---

20 Minutes warm up @ 75% MHR

20 Minutes @ AT heart rate

5 Minutes @ 75% MHR (active recovery)

15 Minutes @ AT heart rate

5 Minutes @ 75% MHR (active recovery)

10 Minutes @ AT heart rate

5 Minutes @ 75% MHR (active recovery)

5 Minutes @ AT heart rate

5 Minutes @ 65% MHR cool down

Run Key Workout #2 – Mile Repeats Running

Building Speed is essential to race preparation if competing is your goal. If you are not feeling the competitive urge for a race, it is not necessary to complete workouts like this one. If you want to be ahead of the field, you CANNOT skimp or miss these intervals. They are simple, time tested, and essential to your program! You'll notice that in the mile intervals, you can choose between 3 to 8 repetitions. It is a good idea to start with 3 and add one or two each week until you reach the number 8. This type of a workout should be done in the 2 months prior to your race.

---

15 minute warm up @ 70% MHR

3 – 8 x 1 mile @ 90-95% MHR with ? the time it took you to finish the last mile as your recovery at 65% MHR.

10 minute cool-down @ 70% MHR

Equipment and Tips

Overhauling the gear closet, what is necessary, what is luxury, what is ludicrous. Running is an eloquently simple sport. The equipment needed is pure and the benefits are astounding. Like anyone driving an old car, however, runners like to dream of the gear that'll "get em there" faster.

Essentials

- Shoes
- Socks
- Carry-along Water Bottle
- Sunscreen
- Hat
- Sun Glasses
- Running Shorts (or Speedo with regular shorts)

Luxury

- Heart Rate Monitor
- Speed / Distance Monitor
- Racing Flats
- Head phones
- More time to run than a 1 hour lunch hour
- Personal Coach
- Training Partner

Ludicrous

- Skinny body

CHAPTER 6

The JULSTRO™ Method of Self-treatment

The Julstro Technique is a deep muscle therapy that grew out of years of treating clients, many of them athletes, with various musculoskeletal injuries. When athletes train they spend hours doing strength movements, contracting the muscles to lift weights, swim, run, cycle, etc. The muscles become overused, and the athlete now has a "repetitive strain injury" that prevents him/her from moving the strained area without pain.

Deep muscle therapy would stop the pain, but the athlete would return to the previous level of exercise, and the problem would come back. I needed to develop a self-treatment system, so that athletes could stop the pain completely, by themselves!

This book will instruct you how to properly self-treat each muscle spasm or contraction. You will become so comfortable with the Julstro Self-Treatments, that you will find your hand automatically going to the correct area whenever you feel a pain in the joint, or in the muscle itself.

While I wouldn't have thought it at the time, I had the "good fortune" of having a lot of painful conditions stop me in my tracks. I didn't know any therapist who could do what I knew needed to be done, so I began to treat myself – and this was the beginning of the Julstro Self-Treatment System. I found that if I could work out a treatment on myself, I could easily teach a client to do the same.

Eventually, as the various methods were developed, I found that teaching my patients how to do the techniques gave them the ability to continue their treatments at home, enhancing the benefits of their office sessions. Since I have joined my practice with Dr. Cohen, the Julstro techniques have been brought to a new level. Throughout this book I will use the pronoun "we" to designate the times when Dr. Cohen was involved. We work together as a team, each adding a piece of expertise that enhances the other, and you receive the benefit of both of us.

There are several advantages to deep muscle therapy: first and foremost, deep therapy brings fresh blood to the muscle, bringing nutrients to the muscle fibers. One of the by-products of muscle action is lactic acid, and when this builds up the muscle is denied access to fresh blood. Our body has a mechanism to release the lactic acid - if we give it enough time. However, modern life keeps us so busy that we keep creating lactic acid, not flushing it away. Working deeply on the muscle is like having a pump for the muscle - when you press down deeply you are pushing the lactic acid out; when you release, blood fills the void.

Deep muscle therapy also stretches the muscle fibers, and releases any contractions or spasms. This allows the joint to move more freely, giving you a better range-of-motion.

When doing the deep movements that are included in the Julstro Technique it is important not to let your fingers (or whatever is providing the pressure) slide on the skin. Did you ever have "rug-burn"? Sliding on the skin while doing deep muscle therapy can cause the skin to have that same feeling.

Prior to treatment, put heat onto the area. Chronic, tight muscles respond well to the comfortable warmth, which will eventually help to release the tightness, making it easier to treat and stretch the muscles.

We also advise people to use a deep-muscle cream, such as Sombra', to help the muscle fibers relax. Put a generous amount on the entire muscle and if possible, place a heating pad over it for 5 minutes prior to doing self-treatment or stretching. You will need to wait until the cream is completely absorbed before you can treat the muscle.

When a muscle is bruised use ice to stop the further bruising. Ice is beneficial when an injury has just occurred within the previous 24 hours. We suggest applying ice after doing any very deep therapy to a muscle. Occasionally deep therapy will bruise fibers, and the day after treatment you may feel like you bumped into a piece of furniture – this is temporary. You may even occasionally see a bruise on your skin. This is not serious, and is no reason for concern, any discomfort goes away in 24-48 hours, and on the plus side, you'll already be moving more easily. When using an ice compress, never put the ice directly on your skin, and never leave it on for more than fifteen minutes at a time. We have also found that arnica gel, which is available at any health food store, is great for healing bruised muscles.

When doing deep muscle therapy we suggest you work each area to your tolerance level. Try to reach for the "hurts so good" level – you'll know it when you reach it! If you don't go deeply enough, you are only treating the surface muscles. You need to apply sufficient pressure to reach the deep muscles. Drink a lot of water after each treatment to help flush away toxins that have been released into your system.

How to Work on Your Own Muscle Spasms

Trigger Points: Spasms, Contractions and Adhesions

The following information will help you learn how to "feel" a trigger point.

Spasms are also known as "trigger points"; the terms will be used interchangeably throughout the book. A spasm of the muscle fibers causes pain, or discomfort, in the muscle or the joint that it is moving.
It is easy to learn how to work on your own muscle spasms. The first thing is to learn how to feel the difference between a spasm, a contraction, and an adhesion.

Healthy muscle feels firm but flexible. Depending on its size it will have hundreds or thousands of fibers lying next to each other in nice straight lines.

Spasms and Trigger Points

A spasm, or Trigger Point, is a knot of muscle fibers that feels like a hard bump in the muscle, like a frozen pea.

To work on a spasm, center your finger – or other source of pressure such as a TP Massage Ball, a dowel, a TP Massage FootBaller, or a rolling pin – directly on top of the spasm, push straight down, pressing for about 30 seconds, and then move an inch or so in either direction. Repeat the treatment. Do this several times in different areas immediately surrounding the spasm. As long as you are not sliding on the skin, you will be doing just fine. Here's a hint; if you find you can't easily glide from one treatment area to the next area, put powder on your hands and rub it in - using oil is not as effective as powder because you will keep slipping as you work deeply on the muscle.

Contractions

A contraction is a shortening of the muscle, and depending on its size or location it feels like a thick rope within the muscle, or the entire muscle may feel thick and hard. To visualize a contraction, think of taking the muscle and pushing the two ends into the center, making the muscle shorter and thicker. The problem is, in our bodies each of the two ends of the muscle is still connected to a bone - and the shortening causes a great deal of tension on the bones. In fact, if the muscle contracts too much it will actually tear from the bone. This is the situation when a person has an Achilles tendon tear at the heel of the foot, shin splints, or a torn hamstring.

To work out a contraction, press down and hold for about 30 seconds, then press down and pull at the same time, going only to the end of the skin's elasticity. Don't slide on the skin. Do this several times. Pick up your fingers just a little, letting the skin release before you put your fingers down again to repeat the movement. This will all be clear as we go through each individual technique. Contractions are also treated easily by using a TP Massage Ball, a dowel, or a TP Massage FootBaller, as shown in the Treatment section of this book.

Another way of treating the muscle is, whenever possible, grip the entire contraction with your whole hand. We tell our clients to grab the muscle as if you were grasping a thick cucumber, and then squeeze it tightly. If you squeeze, and pull at the same time with the intention of lengthening the muscle, you will accomplish flushing and stretching the muscle in one movement.

Do each of these techniques along the entire length of the muscle. You will find that each time you do the movements it will hurt less. This is because the spasms and contractions are lengthening, and the tension is being released from the muscle fibers.

Adhesions

Adhesions are the body's way to protect an injured muscle fiber, and is actually a phenomenon called "splinting". If a fiber gets injured, the muscle puts out a sticky substance that causes the fibers next to the injured fiber to stick, allowing the injured fiber to relax because it is being carried along with the adjoining fibers. This reduces the power of your muscle by taking some of the fibers out of action. Instead of each fiber working independently, giving you the ability to use all the fibers required to do the task you want, the center fibers are not working at all, decreasing your strength.

Adhesions feel like tight strings. To break them down you go across them like you are playing a guitar. Adhesions aren't usually painful; in fact you rarely know they are there. Eventually you will begin to realize that you don't have the power that you once had, and you don't know why.

Having worked with thousands of clients, we have found that in many cases muscles are overlooked when physicians are diagnosing painful joint problems. This is particularly true of carpal tunnel syndrome and low back pain: the muscles in the area are rarely even considered before surgery is planned. Dr. Cohen and I both believe it behooves everyone, prior to having surgery on any joint, as well as back surgery, to first check the muscles that are affecting the joint. The best person to examine the muscle is a massage therapist who does deep tissue therapy, and is fully trained in muscles, their actions, referred pain areas, and the reaction of the body to contractions of the muscle.

While other types of therapies concentrate on ligaments, bones, and the nervous system, deep muscle therapy concentrates solely on the action of muscles on the joints. Massage therapists are trained to use the sensitivity of their hands to find and treat these problems.

Spasm Relief Tools – The Julstro Tool, TP Massage Ball and FootBaller, and Clothes Hanger Poles!

When I began teaching our clients how to treat their own spasms I found that some people had difficulty because of lack of flexibility. In some cases, such as the back, the area couldn't be reached without the aid of a tool, and for other areas strength was a problem. As a result, several simple tools became the method of choice. In this book I'll be showing you how to do the treatments using your own hands and arms, and also using a variety of simple "tools" such as a length of 2" thick dowel (commonly used as a clothes hanger pole in your closet), a door jam, a tennis ball, or a golf ball.

Athletes would tell me that the tennis ball was "too soft, it collapses when I lean on it", and they would try a baseball, but that was too hard. We searched for the right combination of firm, but soft, and finally found it while at the Ironman Lake Placid Competition in July of 2003. The TP Massage Ball is perfect, and it comes with a welcome second "tool" called the TP Massage FootBaller. The "FootBaller" looks like a lightweight dumbbell with the cross-bar made of the same hard/soft material as the Massage Ball. Between these two products we have been able to develop even more techniques than before, and athletes have been thrilled with the results.

We no longer suggest that people use a tennis ball, and we have also eliminated the golf ball from our suggestions on how to treat the feet. Your own body (as shown throughout this book), the two TP Massage tools, and a 24" length of 2" thick dowel (clothes hanger pole) are all that you need to effectively treat all the muscles in your body!

Anyone who purchases the Julstro Video System for the treatment of Carpal Tunnel Syndrome, will also receive a specially designed tool, called the Julstro Tool. This tool has many uses throughout the body. Proper use of the Julstro Tool for the forearm and hand is explained in the video package.

It has been fun working with each client to decide which tool will work best. As we worked closely with serious athletes who compete in 26.2 mile marathons, 100+ mile cycling races, and Ironman competitions, we have found how to do the Julstro Technique "on the run". Dr. Cohen and I appreciate your input - and are happy to be beneficial to you and to your sport!

Specialized Tools

As we mentioned, we have found two tools that are especially useful at doing deep treatment of trigger points, the TP Massage Ball™ and Footballer™, and the companion piece, the TP Baller Block™. Together, these three items, along with the 2" dowel, are all the equipment you'll need to effectively work every spasm in your body.

We asked Cassidy Phillips, the President of Trigger Point Technologies and inventor of the TP Massage Ball, Footballer, and Baller Block to introduce his products to you:

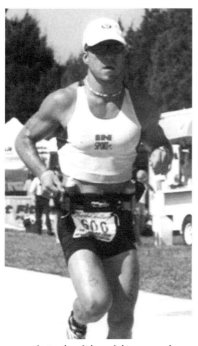

I am Cassidy Phillips, founder of Trigger Point Technologies, LLC. I've been doing triathlons for over twenty years and have had as many injuries as cars on the road. At the age of ten I became addicted to studying biomechanics, trying to make myself the most efficient athlete I possibly could. As the years went by and the training got more intense different pains set in. There wasn't one person I could ask to get the answers I was looking for. What is causing the pain? Just getting out of the bed some mornings to get to the pool was a two-hour ordeal. Three chiropractic appointments and massages throughout the week weren't enough. I was soon diagnosed with fibromyalgia, a chronic disorder associated with widespread muscle and soft tissue pain, tenderness and fatigue. One doctor told me that training at a competitive level was impossible. The news threw me into a depression. That was short-lived because it only motivated me to problem-solve my illness.

After intense research and education from nutritionists, chiropractors, massage therapists, holistic healers, medical doctors and orthopedics, I realized that my solution needed three elements: proper nutrition, plenty of sleep, and massage, later to be defined as a manipulation of trigger points that riddled my body. As an athlete, I was concerned about speed, performance and biomechanics but failed to include proper nutrition and sleep to my regimen. That was the first situation to address.

The second was to research muscular structure, trigger points, and the human body's ability to repair the damage created by toxicity within the center of the muscle. My research also found that loss of dorsiflexion in the foot causes improper biomechanics, causing the common problems that athletes deal with; Plantar Fasciitis, IT Band Syndrome, Piriformis Syndrome and more. This forced me to take that same aggressive approach I took to training and apply it to research and development for the best applications to allow me to achieve what I was learning. This led me to develop a patent-pending material that is used in Trigger Point Technologies: TP Massage Ball™ and TP Massage FootBaller™.

The awesome part about all of this is that my research has changed the lives of so many. Athletes all over the world are achieving more wattage, power and proper biomechanics by using our Trigger Point Technologies devices. By creating the elasticity within the muscle you generate free wattage and power because it is already there, it's just stuck in the scar tissue or muscle spasm due to over use, poor hydration and diet, injury, or just the plain old act of life.

TP Massage Ball™

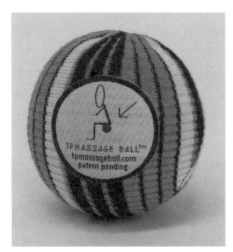

The TP Massage Ball's dense materials mirror the feeling of an actual thumb, changing shape after 5-7 seconds of pressure. This material is superior to other balls, such as a tennis ball which will collapse and only touch the surface of the muscle. The dense, but soft, material penetrates the nucleus (belly) of the muscle safely and effectively.

Whether the **TP Massage Ball** is used on the quads, glutes, hips, piriformis, hamstrings, back or shoulders, the technique remains the same...hold the **TP Massage Ball** in place for 5 to 7 seconds, take a deep breath and then roll. Use the **Ball** for 3 to 5 minutes at any given time before and after a workout, a race and prior to stretching.

TP FootBaller™

Notice how easy the FootBaller is to use. The photo shows how the hands apply an ample amount of pressure. This treatment can be done hands-free with the pressure being applied by using the other foot on top of the leg being treated. As pressure is applied and the user takes a deep breath, the material slightly changes shape in about 5 to 7 seconds penetrating the belly of the muscle. The user should then roll the FootBaller up and down along the length of the muscle and side to side, manipulating the width of the muscle. If the athlete pronates, they may have to bring their leg or knee inward slightly. The smaller the movement, the more concentrated the muscle manipulation. The Baller Block is used to prop the Footballer off the ground to allow it to actually roll and also to guarantee that the foot stays relaxed.

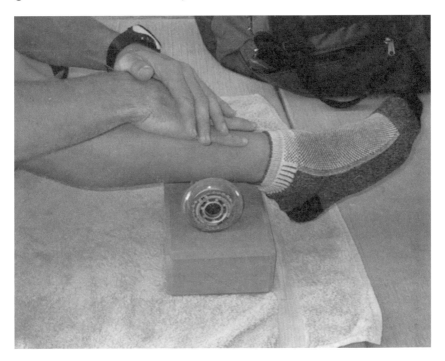

Now we address your Bio-Mechanics

Truth be told, running on a cambered road can cause a fair share of problems, but people sit a lot more than anything else...introducing the **TP Baller Block.** It is designed to retrain the thought process about sitting. When driving in a car, the left knee will brush the side door panel and the foot will turn upward. Comfort is lost and fatigue sets in. Unfortunately, this is the beginning of the whole process. Not only is the soleus compromised and elasticity lost due to the prolonged position of your foot but also the piriformis is jeopardized loosing elasticity because of the angle of the leg.

Place the **TP Baller Block** between the thigh and the door panel (see picture). The placement of the block will not allow the leg to fall to the side towards the door, which produces a more erect posture. This is working on biomechanics while you are not training adding comfort to your everyday life. Keep biomechanics and structural integrity in line throughout your day to prevent discomfort while training and racing.

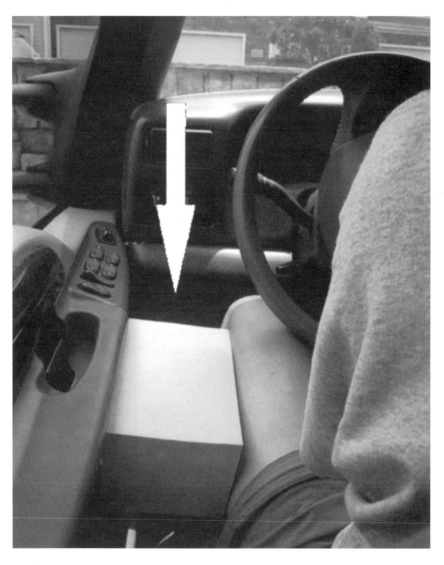

Another innovative way to utilize the **TP Baller Block** is to place the block between the knees or quads and lightly squeeze (see pictures below) or just hold the block in position. This is great while sitting at a desk, on a plane, bus or subway when you don't have a door panel to rest the Baller Block up against. This strengthens the adductors while retraining your thought process to not let your legs bow out to the sides on a regular basis.

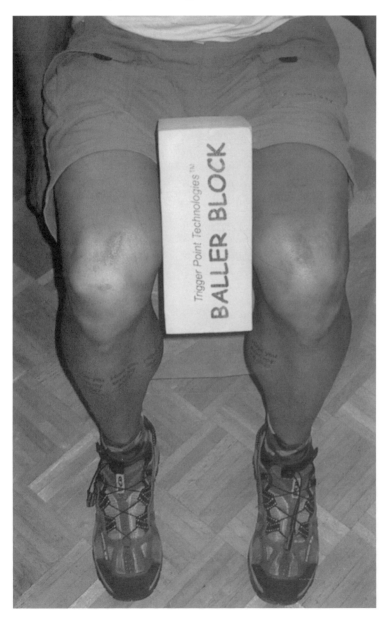

We at Trigger Point Technologies want athletes to understand that they shouldn't have to stop doing what they love just because of pain or discomfort. By attacking the problem, the symptom will be alleviated. Getting a massage isn't the difficult part, getting to the therapist is! With the awesome help of this great book you can finally get the answers you've desired."

Your Gym Bag

You can carry immediate pain-relief in your gym bag! We strongly suggest you add these products, and the dowel, to your work-out bag so you'll have them with you at all times. Pain can stop you in your tracks, but with knowledge and a few light tools, you can eliminate the pain immediately.

The TP Massage Ball, FootBaller and Baller Block can be ordered by going to our website: www.julstro.com, or by copying the order sheet at the back of this book.

When to Use Heat and Cold Packs

Dr. Cohen suggests that the rule of thumb is: cold if the injury is less than 24-36 hours old (called "acute"), and heat when the injury is of longer duration (called "chronic"). Also, if there is considerable pain, regardless of whether the injury is acute or chronic, the cold pack will help to numb the area and give relief.

After doing a strenuous exercise program, or after working deeply on a muscle, always use ice to heal any muscle trauma. Never put ice directly onto the skin, put cloth between the ice and the skin to prevent freezing of the skin tissue. Ice should only be applied for 15 minutes at a time. Let the skin return to body temperature for 15 minutes and then apply again if necessary. If the skin is cold for longer than 15 minutes at a time it can cause damage to the skin and muscles.

The body has an innate intelligence that will tell us whether to use heat or cold. If we imagine putting heat on an area, and then think how it feels, and do the same with imagining cold on the area, we will know our body's answer.

CHAPTER 7

The Trigger Point Charts

Finding the Source of Pain

In Chapter 1 Dr. Cohen explained muscle action and the term "Trigger Point". This book uses colorful trigger point charts, which were drawn by Jerry Trump from the research published by Janet Travell, MD, and David Simon, MD. The charts will to help you find the source of your pain.

The abbreviation "TP" will be used to designate the Trigger Point Charts. The abbreviation "M" will be used to designate the Muscle Charts which have been included for your convenience.

On the TP charts you will see circled "x" marks; these are the trigger points. You will also see areas shaded in the same color. The darker colored area is the primary point of referred pain, and the lighter shaded areas may be involved to a lesser degree. The name of the muscle is printed in the same color as its corresponding area of pain.

When you locate the area where you are feeling pain on the chart, go to the name of the muscle in the caption under the index to find where the treatment for that muscle is located.

An important fact is that the "x" may be so far away from the referred pain area that it is actually on two different figures on the chart! Also, an "x" may be shown on the left, or right, side of the body. We have the same muscles on both sides of our body, and the spasm could be on either side. The chart shows it on only one side so as not to have to be repeated.

The body is extremely predictable. Pain "refers" (is felt) in areas distant from the trigger point: for example, notice on TP Chart 1 that a trigger point in the neck has a pain referral in the chest, the upper back, the entire length of the arm and the hand! This caused us a moment's uncertainty about where we should put the treatment for a trigger point in the neck: should it go in the chest, back, arm, or hand? We decided to always put the treatment in the section where the pain would be felt.

As more and more athletes came to us with sports-related injuries, either through online forums or in the office, we worked together to develop ways for them to do the self-treatments during their training sessions - and even during a competition.

The Muscle Charts have been included to help you understand the text regarding each muscle. You will see the origination and insertion of each muscle, and you will be able to clearly understand how the muscle can cause pain far from the site of the spasm.

One last thought. Muscles have long, and sometimes complicated, Latin names. While it is not necessary for you to learn the names of the muscles, we will use them so you will be able to locate the trigger points on the charts.

PART III
THE JULSTRO TREATMENTS

CHAPTER 8

Upper Body Pain and Tingling

Scalenes: A Very Special Muscle – The Cause of Pain & "Tingling" in the Entire Upper Body!

It was a challenge to decide where to place the scalenes. While they are a neck muscle, they rarely cause neck pain – with one major exception that has been brought to our attention in a testimonial sent to the Carpal Tunnel Treatment Center, which will be discussed further into this chapter.

The scalenes are composed of three muscles: the anterior, the medial, and the posterior scalenes. The origin of the muscle is attached to the front of the 1st and 2nd ribs, and the end point – the insertion – is on the 2nd to 6th cervical vertebrae of the neck.

When the scalenes contract it brings your head down toward your chest.

Think of the millions of times you do this every day and yet the only way to stretch this muscle is a movement that is rarely done – that's where the problem lies!

When a muscle is constantly contracted, and not stretched, it shortens. As mentioned in Chapter 1, a phenomenon called "muscle memory" keeps a contracted muscle at that shortened length. This puts a great strain on the ends of the muscle, especially at the insertion points. Since the insertion points of the scalenes are on the vertebrae of the neck, when the muscle is contracted from a spasm, it pulls the vertebrae out of alignment. As this happens it causes the opposite side of the vertebrae to press deeply onto the spinal cord, and traps the nerves that pass through the vertebrae going to the muscles of the upper body.

The pressure on the spinal cord so close to the skull, as a result of the contracted scalenes (and also the levator scapulae – see Chart 10) is a common cause of severe headaches.

If you examine Chart 1 of the scalenes, you will notice that the "x" pinpointing the spasms are all in the neck, but the shading that represents the referred pain areas are in:
> the back of the head;
> down into the chest;
> down the middle of the back;
> the front and back of the shoulder
> upper arm, and forearm; and, finally
> into the hand!

We guarantee that most medical doctors, or therapists, will not examine your scalenes when you present to their office with wrist or hand pain.

Let's look at the logic behind the scalenes causing such a wide area of pain.

The back of the head: as spasms in the scalenes pull the vertebrae down and forward, your chin moves slightly down toward your chest. This makes the back end of the vertebrae push up. This may be very slight, but over time it will change the curve of your neck, this change can often be seen in an x-ray of the neck. As long as there hasn't been damage to the bones, when you release the spasms you can begin the reverse process and restore the neck to its original curve.

When the scalenes are contracted they also put strain on a series of small muscles called the suboccipital muscles. These muscles hold the vertebrae together, and when they are strained they cause pain around the back and sides of the skull, causing a headache feeling at the base of the skull.

I mentioned in the beginning of this chapter that Dr. Cohen and I received a wonderful testimonial from a gentleman who had purchased the Julstro Video System for Carpal Tunnel Syndrome. He had gotten the Video System because he was experiencing wrist pain and numbness that was preventing him from doing simple movements such as grasping objects, or turning doorknobs.

In 1992 he was diagnosed with bone spurs on the cervical (neck) vertebrae pressing into the cervical disks. The physicians weren't able to do surgery because of the location of the spurs. He was in constant pain and lived on pain medications when he received the Julstro System in the mail.

He wrote to us that "The first time I did the Julstro System, I was practicing the scalenes treatment, while pressing on a spasm the pain shot directly into the area of my neck that had been hurting for years. I could feel that this was possibly the cause of my condition, so I focused with the intention of releasing the spasms . . . and it worked! For the first time in 9 years the pain was gone from my neck! It only took one treatment, and it was gone!" He wrote to us one week later, to tell us that for the last 7 days he had been completely pain free, and was no longer taking the pain medications.

This testimonial made us look even closer at the scalenes, and their involvement in neck pain and headaches.

If you are near a computer, before reading this next section, link to the graphic of the scalenes so you will have it readily available to examine: http://www.aboutcts.com/scalenes.html

The bundle of nerves that passes through the scalenes is called the brachial plexus. These are the nerves that send sensation to the muscles in your upper body and the entire length of your arm and hand. As you look at the way the muscle crosses the nerves, you can understand why a spasm, or contraction, presses the nerves. This pressure disturbs the normal nerve impulse going to the muscles – causing pain, tingling, or numbness.

Common areas of pain that are caused by a scalenes spasm pressing on the brachial plexus are:

- Pressure in the back of the head & neck. When posterior scalenes are pulling down on the vertebrae they cause a tight feeling that radiates around the entire back of the head, and down into the neck. People often described it as a "pressure headache", as if they had a tight band, or cap, on the back of their head.

- Pain and "burning" down into the chest. A common referred pain area is down into the chest, and gives burning pain that can mimic a heart attack.

- The feeling of a razor-blade cutting into the middle of the back, next to the shoulder blade, is another common area of referred pain. We have found that we must release the pressure on the brachial plexus in order to relieve pain in the area of the shoulder blade.

- Pain, numbness, burning, and a feeling of "weakness" in the shoulder, upper arm and forearm are all common sensations when the anterior scalenes are pressing onto the brachial plexus.

- When the scalenes press onto the median nerve as it separates from the brachial plexus, you get numbness, and tingling, in your thumb and first two fingers. This is often misdiagnosed as carpal tunnel syndrome, but the pressure isn't in the carpal tunnel at all – it is in the neck.

The scalenes are involved in many different painful conditions, however, this treatment is a bit more complicated. The treatment is near a major artery and doing it incorrectly may be harmful.

The full scalenes treatment is taught on the Julstro Self-Treatment Video System. We have found that people can easily learn how to do the self-treatment when they watch us demonstrate it, "live" on the video. You can read the testimonials of others who have used the Video System by visiting our website.

To learn how to self-treat the scalenes spasms quickly, releasing trapped nerve fibers, visit our website at: http://www.aboutcts.com.

CHAPTER 9

TMJ – Jaw Pain

We have treated many athletes who have severe jaw pain, and headaches, caused by clenching their teeth while they are working out with weights. Tightly clenching the jaw causes a condition that is commonly called "TMJ", and while it won't hinder your athletic ability, it will cause pain while doing something as simple as eating. It's caused by a strong muscle that closes your jaw as it contracts, and allows you jaw to open when it relaxes. When there is a spasm in the masseter muscle your jaw remains shut, or is extremely painful to open. In fact, if the masseter muscle is totally contracted by a spasm you will have a condition called "lock jaw" and will be advised to have the muscle surgically released. Fortunately, a simple treatment will reverse the problem and alleviate all of the pain.

Put your fingertip onto the spasm and press down. Hold the press for 60 seconds and then, while still pressing on the muscle, slowly open your jaw as far as possible. Do this several times, increasing the pressure on the spasm each time. Then check the muscle to see if there are any other spasms and treat them the same way.

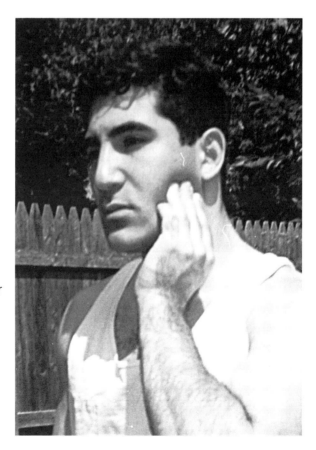

You can very easily stop jaw pain by doing this treatment several times, opening your jaw wider each time you are pressing the muscle.

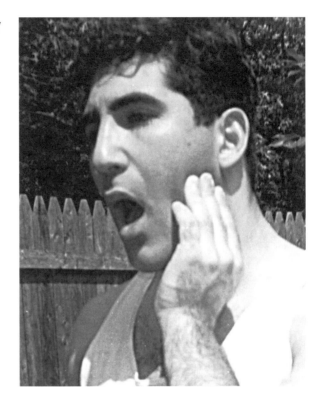

Chapter 10

The Stiff Neck - and Other Neck Pains

Many people get so tight in the upper back and neck muscles that their necks become almost locked in position. Some people call it "stiff neck"; others just complain that they can't look over their shoulders without pain. We turn our heads thousands of times a day, so any stiffness in this area is constantly being noticed.

The muscles of the neck, and the muscles of the shoulder, are so diverse in their actions that they give us an incredibly wide range-of-motion...when all the muscles are working properly! Think of the movements you can do with your head, and neck - up/down, left/right, circle, bend forward & back, tilt in any direction, it's amazing!

For every movement, specific muscle fibers must contract to enable you to move. In order for your head to turn right, the muscles on the left must relax and stretch. If you want to lean your head back, the muscles in the front must stretch. This is true for every movement our bodies make, but muscle spasms can upset this delicate balance!

If you are trying to turn left, but the muscles on the right are contracted, you can't turn. Many therapists tell clients that they need to "strengthen the muscles on the left", but they fail to look at the muscles on the right to see if they are stretching. We have seen thousands of clients whose pain was the result of tight muscles! You need to think, "which muscle should be stretching in order to make this movement", and examine that muscle.

The condition that is commonly called "stiff neck" occurs when all of the muscles - or at least the majority of the muscles - that turn the head in any direction, go into a severe spasm at the same time. The head won't turn in any direction! Since the muscles are exerting a great deal of tension on the bone, the person is usually in a great deal of pain.

Stiff neck is a phenomenon that, fortunately, is relatively rare. While it is common for a person to have neck pain when a muscle is contracted, it is rare when all the muscles contract together, at the same time, creating this severe condition. When this does happen, the person needs to find a trained deep muscle therapist, and also do the Julstro techniques to help speed the process along.

The first thing that needs to be done is to warm up the muscle so that the muscles begin to relax. We suggest using heat for five minutes prior to treatment. Use a large enough heating pad to cover the entire neck and upper shoulders. Moist heat is superior to dry heat.

The Sternocleidomastoid muscle, nicknamed "SCM", is one of the primary causes for stiff neck. This muscle has lots of pain referral points, all in the head, and NONE in the neck. Most people are surprised when they find how painful this muscle can be - and the relief that treating it offers!

Look at Chart 18 to see the areas of pain that originate in the SCM. The long Latin name for the muscle is Sternocleidomastoid - a handful to say - but it means it originates on the sternum and the clavicle (commonly called the breastbone and the collarbone), and inserts on the mastoid (a bone just behind the ear). It refers pain to the ear, and is frequently the cause of tinnitis (ringing in the ears), loss of equilibrium, and ear pain. The referral to the eyes can mimic a sinus headache, or eyestrain, and there is an area of referred pain that wraps around the skull and gives a throbbing headache.

Two interesting clients who proved the impact of a contracted SCM were exceptional because they had pain in areas that would never lead a physician to look at a neck muscle. The first patient was experiencing numbness in the side of her face, a symptom that mimicked Bell's Palsy. After a complete medical workup, her physicians were unable to find the cause of her condition. As it turned out a severely contracted SCM was the culprit. It took only one deep muscle treatment for the numbness to begin to fade, and by the end of the second treatment, she had full sensation back in her face.

The second was a man with tinnitis. He had been suffering for 3 weeks with constant ringing in his right ear, telling us "it's driving me crazy – it never stops!" He had been sent for the full battery of tests to check for some very serious causes of the ringing, which were all normal. After only a few minutes into the self-treatment for the SCM the ringing began to subside, and by the end of the session he was 100% better. It was because of this client that we realized how frequently pain, and ringing, in the ear is caused by SCM contractions. As is often the case, muscle contractions can cause many different conditions. If the underlying muscle spasm is not properly treated the condition will generally not go away on its own.

While it's a bit tricky to catch hold of the SCM muscle, if you follow the sequence of pictures shown, you should be able to do it just fine. Once you've found it, you'll always be able to easily do it again.

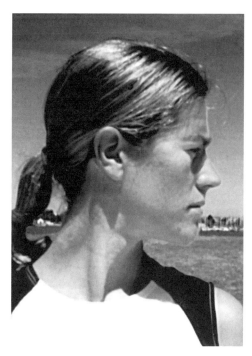

To catch the SCM turn your head all the way to the side, going as far as you can go and really stretching as if to look over your shoulder. Now, feel the side of your neck and you will find a muscle that goes from the back of your ear to the center of your collarbone. That is the SCM.

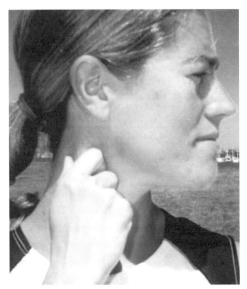

Next, take the first two joints of your same side pointer finger and the flat of your thumb to pinch the muscle. Once you have your thumb on one side, and the first two joints of your pointer finger on the other side of the SCM, turn your head to face forward. Now apply pressure to the muscle by squeezing your thumb and finger together.

It is important to avoid the carotid artery, which is found at the bottom half of your neck, toward the front. If you feel a pulse between your fingers, you are holding the artery, just move up 1-2" and you will be ok.

Go as close to your ear as you can, since that is where most of the problems originate. This area is above the carotid artery, and it is safe to treat. Hold the pinch for about 30 seconds and then move either up or down a bit, and repeat treatment.

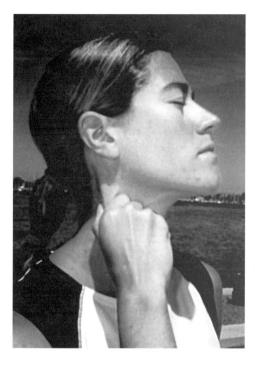

After you have worked on the muscle for a minute or more, continue holding the pinch and then slightly pull your head back at an angle away from your hand. This will stretch the muscle.

To complete the treatment of the SCM, run your fingertips firmly across the middle of your collarbone, at the area directly under your jaw line. If you feel bumps, pain, or tightness, just work them out by centering your fingertip right onto the bump, and then rubbing it firmly along the bone.

The Back of the Neck and Headaches

The back of your neck is actually the beginning of the muscles in your upper back. Most of the muscles that originate here travel down your shoulders and upper back, spasms in this area are a major cause for tightness in the neck. When a person has limited range-of-motion in the neck, we always look at the back first. We suggest you do all the back treatments first, and then move up to the neck treatments.

The muscles of the upper back and neck are primary to the relief of tension headaches. If you suffer with tension headaches these treatments, done on a regular basis, will be of great benefit. If you are having a headache, the treatment will reduce the intensity almost immediately. In the case of severe tension headaches, we have found that clients can successfully decrease the intensity of the headache by themselves, but they need to have a course of deep-muscle treatments for the pain to disappear completely.

Cycling is a primary cause of contracted muscles in the back of the neck. When an athlete is riding in the aerodynamic position they are bent all the way over at the waist and need to bring their head back in order to see the road before them. Contracting the muscles for several hours will elicit "muscle memory" and will cause all of the posterior neck muscles to shorten.

There are so many muscles in the back of your neck that we will be giving you general directions.

Although you will naturally do both sides of your neck, to make explanation easier, we'll be describing how to work on the left side of the neck, using the right hand. This is actually a continuation of the upper back and shoulder treatments. If you read the directions regarding your shoulder in the following chapter, it will make this treatment easier to do.

It will help you understand the impact that the muscles are having if you look at the muscles that are being discussed: splenius cervicis, multifidus, splenius capitis, suboccipitals, levator scapulae, upper trapezius and erector spinae. Also, each muscle is on a different referred pain chart - to see the areas of referred pain, look at Chart 6, Chart 10, and Chart 20.

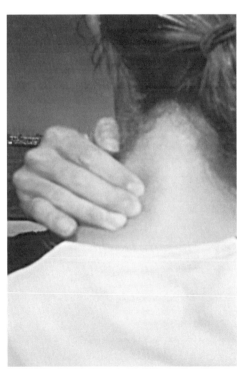

Bring your right arm across the front of your body, placing the three middle fingers of your right hand onto the muscles just left of your cervical vertebrae. With your right fingers crooked, and your arm at an angle from your body, move your middle fingers up the back of the neck.

If you "walk" up the muscles, using deep pressure, you can find the spasms easily. If it hurts when you press on a spot, you've found a spasm. To treat it, just put your middle finger right onto the point, and pull your elbow out from your body, and then down toward the floor.

Remember, all strength comes from your arm, not from your hand.

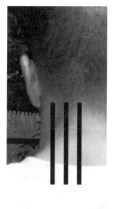

Go all the way from your shoulder junction up to your skull. Make three "lines"; the first will be right next to your spine, then 1" to the left, and then again 1" further to the left.

If you feel something that is like a slippery rope sliding under your fingers, know that it is a contracted muscle. Normally it shouldn't feel like that, and your goal is to flatten and lengthen it. You can do that by centering onto the muscle, pressing deeply in on it, and then pulling your fingers down toward the floor WITHOUT sliding on your skin.

To increase the stretch of the muscle you can drop your head directly down toward your chest while you are pressing the muscle, and slightly turn your chin toward the opposite shoulder. Remember that you want to do a 60-second stretch, so try to hold each point for 10-15 seconds. When you are finished, shake out your shoulders and neck by moving drawing your shoulders up and then dropping them while you are turning your head. By the way, if you hear little crackling sounds in your neck, don't worry. It's called "crepitus", caused by little air pockets being released from muscle fibers - sort of like popping little air-filled "bubble wrap" bumps. The next important movement is a bit tricky but, with practice, you'll do just fine. When a person is having a headache this muscle is very pronounced and easy to grasp.

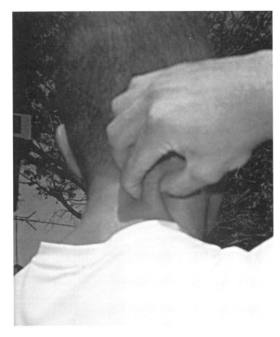

To grab this muscle tilt your head back, relax, put your fingertips directly over your spine, and put your thumb about 3" out from the spine. In between you will feel a tight rope of muscle. Grip it as firmly as you can. You'll find it's quite painful, especially if you are experiencing a headache.

Stay within your own tolerance level, but do grip with good pressure. The closer to your scalp you can grip, the faster your headache will subside. If you focus your attention on the muscles that are just to the side of the cervical vertebre you can treat four important muscles of the neck: upper trapezius, levator scapulae, splenius capitis and splenius cervicus.

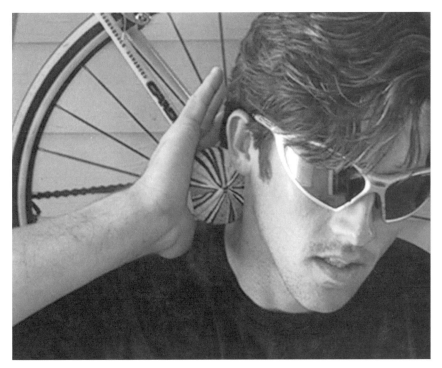

Two methods that work deeply on the posterior neck muscles are by using the TP Massage Ball (shown above) or the dowel (shown below). Be careful not to press on the vertebre and only use enough strength to cause a "feels so good" pressure on the muscles.

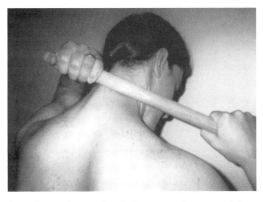

To enhance the movement you can slowly drop your chin to your chest and draw your shoulders down while you are pressing on the neck muscles.

With all of the above Julstro self-treatments, while you are pressing, or gripping, move your head until you feel the muscle stretching – this will hasten the benefits of the treatments.

Headaches take a long time to go away completely, but you should be able to bring some relief after just a few minutes.

CHAPTER 11

The Shoulders, the Upper Back and Headaches

There are several causes for pain in the shoulder, surprisingly – a major one is a neck muscle – the scalenes. Chapter 8 discusses the scalene muscles and how to treat them successfully. We recommend that you examine that treatment when you are looking for the source of shoulder pain.

It is common for people to tell us "I hold all my stress in my shoulders and upper back". Tightness in the shoulder and chest causes round shoulders, stretching them will improve posture. We have seen many clients who suffer from severe headaches get relief by simply releasing the spasms in the upper back and shoulders. Self-treatment is tricky in this area. However with a bit of practice it can easily be accomplished.

One of the interesting things about shoulder pain is that most of the time the pain is coming from someplace not near the shoulder, and in one case pain in the front of the shoulder is actually coming from the back of the body!

It was because of shoulder pain that we first met Jerry Trump, the Ironman Triathlete who wrote the Foreword of this book. To compete in the Ironman Triathlon, a person spends many hours every day running, cycling, swimming and lifting weights. Jerry had a goal, one that he dreamed about, and planned, for many years. When he was only a few months away from his first Ironman, he experienced two pains that, untreated, would put an end to his dream. The most serious was Achilles tendonitis, the second, while less serious would have cut down his speed enough to threaten his not finishing the race in the time allowed. It was a sharp pain in the front of his shoulder that was being called rotator cuff injury, bursitis, or tendonitis.

Physical therapy wasn't helping; anti-inflammatory drugs weren't helping, so Jerry was learning how to "live with the pain". He was determined to race!

I met Jerry "online". He's a beautiful artist and we discussed his sculptures and paintings. When he learned what I did for a living, he asked about his shoulder pain. Several emails, and a few questions, later I knew that Jerry was suffering from the pain of a contracted infraspinatus muscle. When you look at Chart 3, you will see that while the muscle is in the back of the shoulder (on top of your shoulder blade), the pain is felt around the cap of the shoulder, down the biceps and deltoid muscles, and down toward the hand.

Jerry quickly learned how to do the Julstro treatment using a tennis ball to work on the muscle. I told him "it will feel like a rope". His next email back had the subject line "Ouch, Ouch, Ouch!" – he had found the muscle! He said: "It doesn't feel like a rope, it feels like the tow line for the QE II". That was when I learned that Jerry wasn't just an artist, he was a serious athlete and the muscle was hindering his swimming.

Jerry is in excellent shape and his muscles are strong. The tennis ball became too soft because it would flatten as he pressed deeply into it. He next tried a baseball which stays firm, but caused bruising because it was so hard. When we found the TP Massage Ball he began to do the treatments with it and he was amazed at the difference this change made. He was able to work deeper than with the tennis ball and without bruising himself as he had when he tried to use a baseball.

One of the problems with the infraspinatus is that it is difficult, if not impossible, to stretch. The only way to lengthen the muscle is with direct pressure on the length of the muscle fibers.

The Infraspinatus

The infraspinatus muscle lies on the lower 2/3 of your shoulder blade (scapula). Pain is referred from the area of the spasm to the area of the insertion. Since the infraspinatus inserts onto the shoulder, that is where you will feel the pain. Because of nerve involvement, the pain spreads to areas far from the muscle; however, you will only find relief from the pain when you go to the source – the trigger point deep in the muscle.

Feel all around the muscle, as far as you can reach. A spasm always hurts to the touch. Many people feel "if it's hurting, leave it alone", but the opposite is actually what you should be doing. If it hurts, work it out!

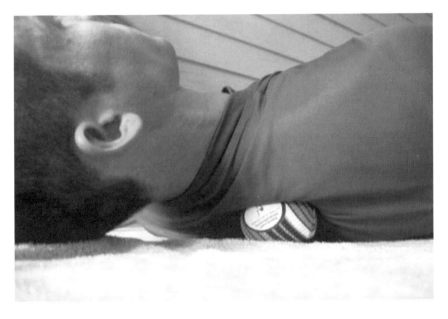

To reach the infraspinatus you will need a TP Massage Ball. Lie on your back on the floor, or on a bed. Put the ball directly onto the muscle, then allow your weight to press the ball into the infraspinatus muscle, moving your body around to maneuver the ball to go along the entire length of the muscle.

Try to go in the direction of the muscle, basically from the lower part of the shoulder blade up toward the point of the shoulder. If you have a contraction in this muscle, it will be quite painful to initially work on it. Gently lean into the ball, only adding more weight as you feel comfortable. The pressure should always be tolerable. It may take you a few treatments to ease the contractions but, with determination, you will succeed!

There is also one muscle that not only causes shoulder pain, but is also a key factor to severe headaches – that muscle is the levator scapula. Look at Chart 10 to locate the levator scapulae, and see the referred pain area of this muscle. Tightness in the shoulder and chest causes round shoulders, so stretching the shoulder muscles will improve posture. Stretching the neck and shoulder first will help when you are treating each muscle spasm.

The first stretch is excellent for the back of your neck, your shoulders, your upper back, and since it stretches the levator scapulae, it may even relieve headaches! This is a multi-bonus stretch because it affects the trapezius muscle from your head all the way down to the middle of your back, and across the shoulders. While you're doing this stretch you will also be affecting the erector spinae, another long muscle that goes from your scalp, down the spine, to just below your waist. Pretty impressive for just one stretch! We suggest warming up the shoulders and upper back by simply rotating the shoulders, circling your head, and slowly moving your entire upper body for a minute or two.

It's best to do this stretch in front of a mirror the first few times. It is very easy to raise the shoulders without realizing it, and therefore not be getting the stretch that you want.

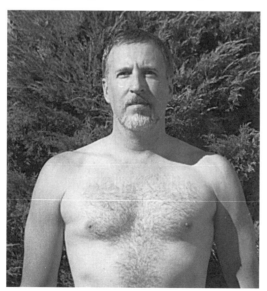

Begin by standing straight with your arms at your side. Imagine you are holding a 50-pound suitcase in each hand. Keep your shoulders level, and don't slouch. Really p-u-l-l your shoulders down toward the floor.

Are your shoulders level, or is one higher? If one is higher, pull that one even more until you look balanced in the mirror.

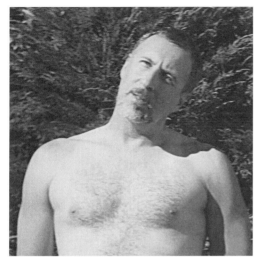

Next, drop your head to the left as if you were trying to touch your left ear to your shoulder, watching in the mirror to ensure that your right shoulder stays down. Do you feel the stretch? Hold that position for about 15 seconds.

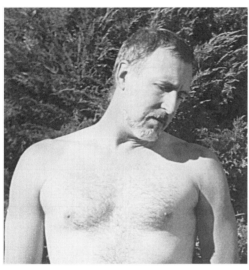

Now, very slowly turn your head.

Remember to pay attention to the position of your shoulders. Your nose will be pointing at your shoulder. You should be able to feel how the stretch changes as you are slowly turning your head. You are stretching all the fibers of the trapezius muscle, as well as the splenius cervicis, the levator scapulae & the multifidus.

Hold the stretch for 60 seconds; next repeat the stretch on the opposite side of your body.

The Trapezius

The trapezius muscle goes from the base of your skull to the shoulder, and then all the way down to the middle of your back. When a therapist is discussing the muscle we divide it into three sections: upper, middle and lower trapezius. The stretch shown above will enable you to feel wherever it is tight along the length of the trapezius muscle.

As you do this stretch you again will need to hold it a full 60 seconds, but when you slowly turn your head during that time you will be stretching all the various fibers of the muscles mentioned above. After doing the stretch on the left side, repeat the stretch on the right side.

After you have done this 2-3 times in front of the mirror you will be able to do it anywhere. You will know when your shoulders are raising, and you'll be able to correct it without looking at them. After each stretch, shake your shoulders out and relax for a few moments.

After completing the stretch your muscles are now ready to do the Julstro treatments. Stand in front of a mirror the first few times, and remember to keep your shoulders as level as possible.

The shoulders and the upper back are tricky for self-treatment; simply because so much of the area is out of our reach. There are several ways we have worked out this problem.

We'll be demonstrating on the left side, using the right hand as the working hand.

Put your right hand on your left shoulder at the point where the shoulder and neck meet. It helps if you place it so your thumb and pointer fingers are on your neck, and the middle finger is the working finger and is right on the junction, just a bit toward the back. Your four fingers should be crooked at each joint of the hand, and your

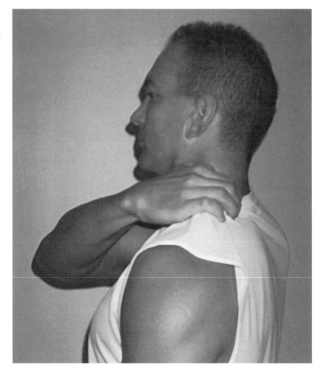

palm should be flat against your body.

Stay in the same spot; relax your arm, with your elbow close to the middle of your chest. In this position you will probably have your middle finger directly on the spasm point.

All the strength from this move is coming from your upper arm, NOT from your fingers. To do that you will simply make sure that your middle finger is on the sore spot, and then pull

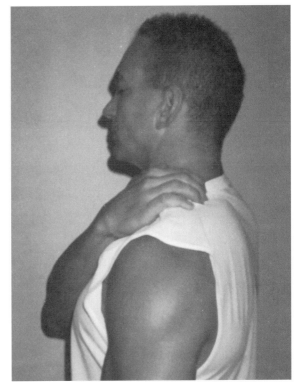

your elbow down toward the floor. Your finger will be like a hook that presses into the spasm.

If you feel your fingers getting tired you are using the hand to give strength, and not your arm. Once you feel the difference it will be easy to do again.

After you have found the trigger point, and you are adding pressure to it, continue pressing into the spasm and do the stretch you just learned for the trapezius muscle.

Hold your shoulders level and drop your head in the opposite direction, rotating your head a bit so your ear is angled toward the front of your chest. By doing this you'll be adding additional stretch to the trigger point, and be releasing it at the same time. Hold this for 15 seconds, and release the pressure. Then do it again, three more times, holding each stretch for 15 seconds.

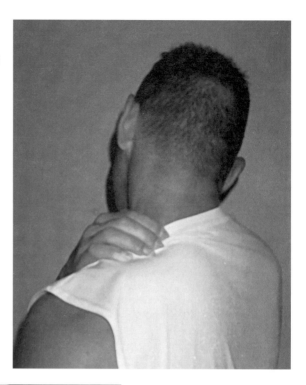

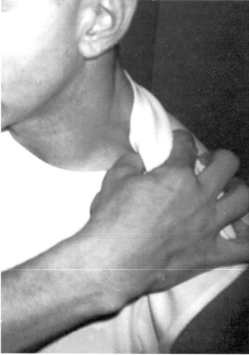

Bring your head up, keeping your hand in the same spot, still pressing on the spasm, take your thumb, flip over onto the front of your shoulder, and push it straight into the muscle. This will move your thumb to a place that will now cause you to be pinching the knot.

You'll feel if you have it right. You should have a fairly thick piece of muscle between the middle finger and the thumb. You can inch your 3 middle fingers back a bit if you find you aren't gripping the entire border of the muscle. Grip tightly and release. Do this four times, for 15 seconds each time. Then shake out your shoulders.

The Supraspinatus

Pain in your shoulder can also be coming from a muscle that is on top of your shoulder blade (scapula). If you look at Chart 10 you will see the pain referral area for the supraspinatus.

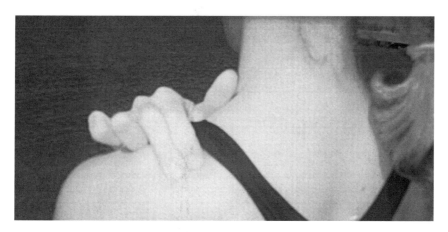

For demonstration purposes, work on the left shoulder, using the right fingers to find the spot. To find the proper spot place your right finger over the top of the left shoulder. Have your fingertips on the top of the shoulder blade. Now, move your shoulder up and down, without moving the left elbow. You will need to use just the muscles of the shoulder to do that, not the muscles of your left arm. Press around into the top of the bone, until you feel a little "gully". If there is a spasm you will feel pain as you press into the muscle. If it hurts, you've found the right spot, and you will be able to easily press out the spasm.

Feel for your shoulder blade with your fingers. When you find the bone, come up a little and you will feel the supraspinatus muscle.

Press your finger directly onto the muscle, and drop your elbow down. The most important thing to remember here is to keep the elbow of your working arm from getting strained.

The shoulder also includes the deltoid muscle. This is the muscle that forms the cap at the top of your arm. If you grab yourself just below the bony point of your shoulder your fingers will be right around the deltoid muscle. This important muscle moves your arm forward, backward, and away from your body. Weight lifters, or anyone doing a repetitive movement while working with weight, or doing heavy lifting, can cause this muscle to become sore.

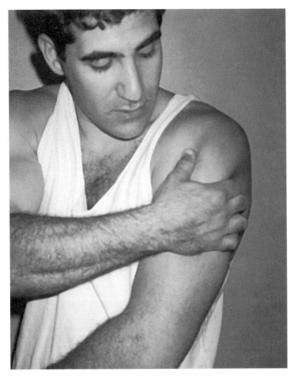

Place your hand around the deltoid muscle, and squeeze it tightly between your thumb and fingers. While squeezing the muscle pull the elbow of your working arm toward the floor and away from the body.

After you have worked on all the spasms on your upper back and shoulder, you can move to the spasms on the front of your body that cause shoulder pain.

Pectoralis Minor and Pectoralis Major

Another muscle that causes shoulder pain is located in your chest. As you look at the graphic of the pectoralis minor muscle, also called "pecs minor", you will see that it originates on your ribcage, and then inserts into a piece of your shoulder blade, called the coracoid process.

The common pain referral area for a spasm in the pecs minor is the entire shoulder cap, and by referral the pain can go all the way down your arm and into your hand. A spasm in this muscle will pull the shoulder forward, as a result this is a primary muscle causing a person to have poor posture and rounded shoulders.

110

Most people don't think of a chest muscle as causing shoulder pain, however, many clients often only get pain relief when spasms are worked out of the pecs minor, and the muscle is stretched properly. To make the instructions easy to follow we will demonstrate this technique on the left pecs minor muscle.

To locate the muscle place your right hand on your chest with your fingers pointing toward your shoulder.

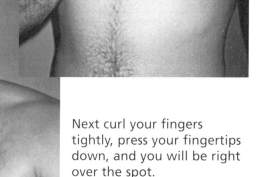

Next curl your fingers tightly, press your fingertips down, and you will be right over the spot.

You can enhance your strength by placing your left hand on top of your right fingers, and press down. Hold the pressure for 15-30 seconds.

While still holding the pressure, bring your left arm up and back, as if going to throw a ball, or do a swimming backstroke. You will feel the muscle stretch as your arm is circling to the back. Continue to make a full circle by going all the way back, down, to the front, and then circle up, back, and around again. Do this 3-4 times. Try to keep your body facing forward while you do this stretch.

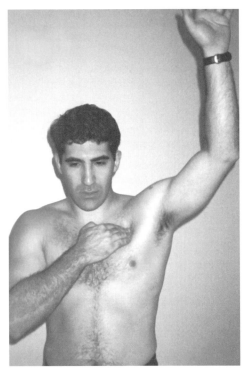

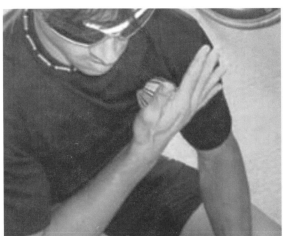

You can also treat the pecs by placing the TP Massage Ball directly on top of the muscle and by pressing down with your opposite hand, roll the ball up toward your shoulder, or...

for the deepest treatment, position the ball between a door jam and your chest and press your body into it, moving your body so the ball rolls up toward your shoulder.

Two other muscles that cause shoulder pain are the Teres Minor and Teres Major. You can treat them, and the pecs, all at the same time with this easy movement.

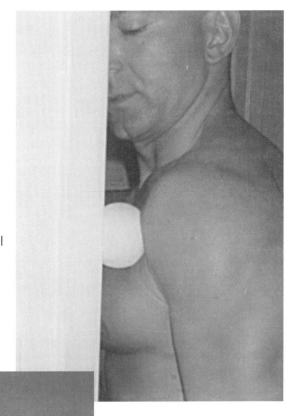

A good way of treating all four muscles is to put your three fingers deeply into your armpit, and put your thumb on the top of the muscle, and squeeze tight. You should be gripping a thick piece of the pectoralis major, and pectoralis minor muscles as well as the teres minor and major muscles.

If you grip a little further toward the top of your arm, you will also be able to treat some of the anterior portion of the Deltoid muscle. After you have a good grip on the muscle, hold it for 60 seconds, and then stretch it by pulling down on it – do not slide on the muscle – maintain your grip and at the same time slightly rotate your arm up and back. You'll feel the muscles stretching as you try, however, if you are gripping the muscle tightly you won't be able to go far with the movement.

If you look at Chart 7 – Pectoralis Minor, as well as Chart 8 - Anterior Deltoid and Pectoralis Major, you will notice that all the trigger points are very close together. As a result you will get a great deal of relief from making minor location changes as you do these self-treatments.

Subclavius

Also, look at Chart 9 - the subclavius muscle, which is located directly under your collarbone (clavicle). This muscle inserts close to the point of your shoulder, and even though it isn't a shoulder muscle, it causes pain to be felt across the front of the shoulder, and down into the biceps muscle.

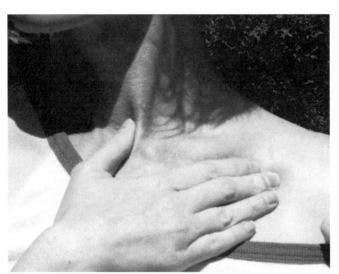

The self-treatment for the subclavius is simply to press your fingers into the muscle, locating the painful area, holding the press for 60 seconds.

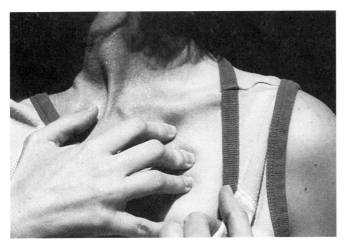

If you feel adventurous you can poke around and find other spasms in the chest, and treat them the same way. Be creative – your intention is to spread the fibers, press them down and lengthen them. Do it in whatever manner seems appropriate to you; just remember to use sufficient pressure to effect a change – light pressure feels nice, but it won't change the length of a muscle fiber. It's nice to know that there is no "wrong" way of doing this treatment, just "effective" or "less-effective" ways. Also, practice makes perfect!

CHAPTER 12

The Arm, Wrist and Hand

The Upper Arm: Biceps and Triceps

The upper arm is composed of two muscle groups, the biceps and the triceps. These muscles give strength to the arm and move the elbow. The deltoid muscle, while actually a shoulder muscle, inserts onto the upper arm and spasms in the deltoid will be felt at the lateral and posterior shoulder and along the upper arm on the inside border.

The biceps consist of one muscle that has two origination points. The long head of the biceps originates on the top of the shoulder, under the border of the shoulder blade. The short head of the biceps originates on a portion of the shoulder blade called the coracoid process. Both of the heads merge into a common muscle belly and insert just below the bend of the elbow, onto the radius, one of the forearm bones.

Because of its origination on the coracoid process, the biceps are frequently also responsible for pressure on the median nerve and the axillary artery. This causes loss of sensation to the arm and hand, as well as diminished circulation to the limb.

When the biceps contract you bend your arm at the elbow. However, when they are in spasm they are pulling on the insertion point, and you feel pain on the inside of your elbow, or at the front of your shoulder (see Chart #2).

Spasms in the biceps are common problems for weightlifters, and swimmers will frequently feel the pain while trying to stretch their arm out fully to take a stroke. When the muscle stays in the contracted position due to a muscle spasm, you cannot open your arm all the way. This will prevent swimmers, tennis and basketball players from using their arms fully, and can even be the cause of having to stop playing the sport.

The treatments are easy, and you can use your arm as leverage to increase the stretch while you are treating the spasm.

There is a point on the biceps that is immediately above the inside of your elbow that refers pain to the wrist and hand. This is a very easy spot to work; all you need to do is cross your arms to find the right location. To demonstrate, use your right thumb to work on your left biceps.

With your arms crossed, place your palms facing down. Have the left arm on the bottom and your right arm on top of it. Your right thumb will be in the perfect position, pointing directly into the bend of the elbow.

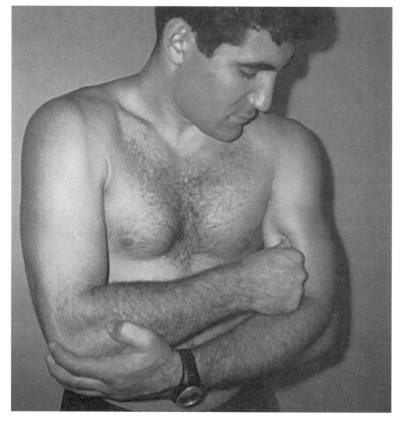

Grip your left upper arm, and press the flat part of your thumb right into the spot. Press around to be sure you are on the center of the spasm, then push into the muscle with your thumb.

Once you find it, apply deep pressure by pushing your entire right arm in toward the spot – don't have the pressure coming just from your hand or thumb, but coming from the right elbow. Keep your wrist straight, without a bend at the joint.

Next you'll want to check out the center (belly) of the muscle.

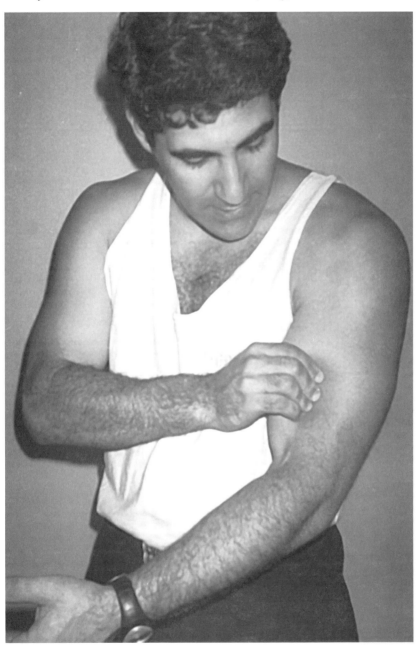

To do that, bend your arm close to your body and put your thumb on the inside of the biceps, and your four fingertips on the outside. Then squeeze all the way in toward the bone, sliding a bit to really grip the fullness of the muscle. This is one of the "hurts so good" areas. Your intention should be to squeeze and pull the muscle away from the bone.

While you are squeezing, slowly open your arm fully. This will increase the stretch given to the muscle. After your arm is out straight, keep your fingers in the same place but release your grip. Bend your arm again, and then repeat the movement. Do this several times.

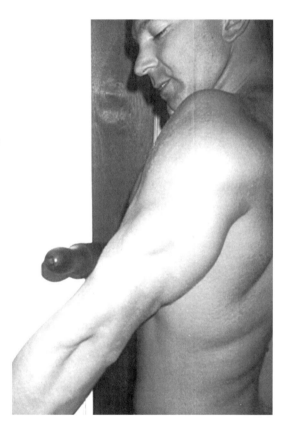

You can also treat the biceps by resting your arm flat against a doorframe and placing a dowel, or a rolling pin, at an angle that will cause pressure on the muscle as you move your body up, causing the dowel to roll down your biceps.

Lean your body forward, and press deeply onto the biceps. All pressure should be going down, toward the hand. When you feel a bump – and it will hurt – that is the spasm that is causing the pain. As you press on the muscle you will be flattening it and pressing out lactic acid.

Triceps Contraction – a.k.a. "Tennis Elbow"

The triceps have three heads, thus the name "triceps". They are located at the back of the upper arm and originate on the posterior/top of the bone, and also on the outer portion of the shoulder blade. Their common insertion point is just below the point of the elbow. When the triceps contract you open your arm from the bent position.

When the triceps are held contracted by a spasm you will have pain at the point of your elbow and you are told you have either tennis elbow, or tendonitis. Often people are told to stop playing their sport, but the following treatments will enable you to continue playing while you are working out the spasms.

The triceps take some time before they are completely healed, but you will feel immediate relief by pressing out the lactic acid that has built up in the fibers, and by stretching the muscle toward the elbow.

Spasms in the triceps cause pain across the entire posterior upper arm, and down into the elbow (see Chart #4).

The position to find the triceps is the same as for the biceps, except you will move the two elbows closer together.

Cross your arms so that your right middle and ring fingers reach all the way around the arm. Deeply press into the muscle. A contraction here frequently feels like a thick rope that goes from the shoulder to the elbow, with the tightest part just above the elbow.

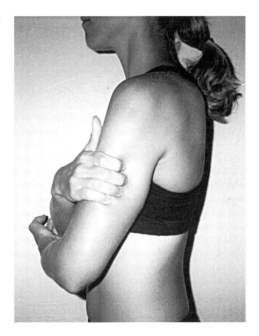

When you find it, try to center your fingers directly on top of the "rope". You may slide over the side of the rope, but keep trying and eventually you will get your fingers to line on top of the fibers.

You can very easily treat the triceps by using the TP Massage FootBaller. Sit at a table and place the TP Massage FootBaller on the tabletop. Bend your arm and place your triceps into the center of the FootBaller. Press down with your arm and then move your 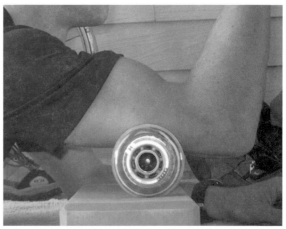 body back and forth to deeply press down along the entire length of the fibers. Put more pressure on the muscle as you move from the top of your arm going toward the elbow, and less pressure as you return to the top of the arm.

Lower Arm, Wrist and Hand – Extension of Forearm Muscles

Repetitive Strain Injury (RSI) as the name implies, develops when a muscle is used over and over again, in the same manner. Eventually the muscle fibers become strained, and shortened, resulting in pain, numbness and loss of flexibility to the areas involved.

As mentioned in Chapter two, when a muscle contracts the opposing muscle must relax. This was demonstrated by using the biceps and triceps, and it is also clearly evident when one looks at the flexors and extensors.

The flexors are on the underside of your forearm and they insert at the wrist, the palm and the fingertips. When they contract you close your hand into a fist and/or curl your hand in toward your wrist.

The extensors are on the top of your arm and insert into the top of the hand and the fingertips, just beneath your fingernails. When the extensors contract you open your closed fist and/or draw your fingers back toward the top of your arm.

The way a muscle moves a joint is like a pulley system. One side contracts, and the other side relaxes. When the forearm muscles contract, your wrist bends and the hand is pulled in that direction. To reverse this, the muscles must relax while the opposing muscle group contracts. Imagine what happens if the relaxing muscle doesn't relax. Your hand locks, and if you force it to move, your wrist will hurt!

The forearms have two main muscle groups, the flexors and extensors. The flexors are on the underside of the arm, and when they contract your hand curls into a fist and/or your wrist bends in toward your arm. The extensors are on the top of your forearm. When they contract your fingers straighten, and/or your wrist bends back & pulls your hand up.

We have seen many athletes who play any sport that involves keeping a closed hand, such as cycling, tennis, or lifting weights, and athletes who are pushing strongly with an open hand, such as swimming, volleyball or basketball, suffer from wrist pain or a feeling of weakness.

The wrist pain occurs because the tight muscle is putting pressure on the insertion point, and you feel pain as the tendon pulls on the bone. The feeling of weakness occurs because the muscle is already shortened by the spasm so it doesn't have its full length to pull on your hand. In order for any muscle to be strong it must be able to stretch to its longest length and then pull from that position. The tighter it is at the start of the movement, the less strength it will have to complete the movement.

As with all the muscles the excess lactic acid must be eliminated and blood must fill the void to nourish the muscle fibers.

This is easy to accomplish by using the TP Massage FootBaller. Sit at a table, or on the floor, and place the FootBaller at a level where you will be able to comfortably place your forearm into it and be able to press down by using your body weight. You may need to use the Block that comes with the FootBaller to bring it up to a comfortable position for you.

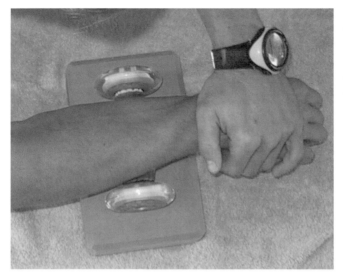

You can treat the flexors by having your palm facing toward the floor.

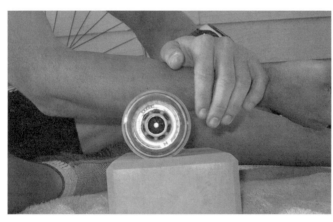

Treat the extensors by having your palm facing toward the ceiling.

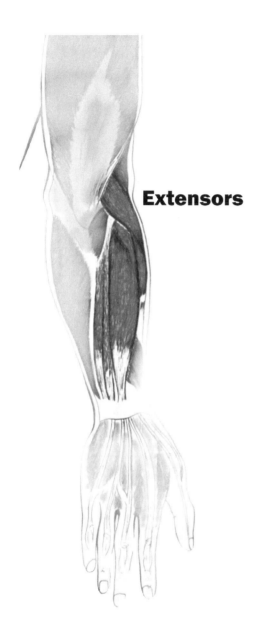

Extensors

To stretch the extensor muscles, put your right arm straight out from the body, with the palm facing the floor. Place your left thumb directly into the bend of your right wrist, and put your left four fingers onto the back of your right hand (not the fingers).

Press down hard, as if you were trying to bend your right hand in the direction of your wrist. Hold this stretch for 60 seconds. Always stay within your comfort zone.

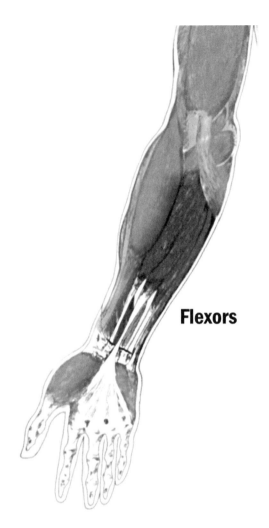

Flexors

To stretch the flexor muscles, you may rest your arm on a table. Holding your arm out straight, and then using the fingers of the opposite hand, gently bend your fingers back. Hold this stretch for 60 seconds.

When you have done the stretches, shake out your hand to get the blood flowing and the muscles relaxed.

CHAPTER 13

The Back

Have you ever had back pain? The odds are very high that your answer is "yes". There are so many things that can happen to cause back pain that entire books have been dedicated to its treatment – and still the search goes on.

All back pain has some connection to the spine, however it is important to understand that the bones of the spine only move because muscles are pulling on them! Unless you have been involved in an accident that forcefully moves a bone out of alignment, the only way for a bone to move is at the direction of a muscle. It is imperative that the muscles are stretched, free of spasms, and functioning properly if the spine is to be aligned properly.

The spine is composed of seven vertebrae in the neck (cervical), twelve in the mid-back (thoracic) and five in the low back (lumbar) region. There are many muscles that insert onto these vertebrae, causing them to move, however, in this book we'll just discuss the major muscles that can be self-treated. Fortunately, all the muscles cross over each other, so when you are working on one muscle group, you are also working on others at the same time.

The use of muscles as "pulleys" is clearly demonstrated as we discuss the back. Have you ever played the game "tug of war"? When I was young we would tie a stick in the middle of the rope, draw a line in the dirt, and put the stick right on the line. Then we drew a big circle, and several of us got on either side of the rope. In order to win your team had to pull the stick over the edge of the circle on your side. We all pulled with all the strength we had, and sometimes we even pulled the other team over the line!

This is a perfect analogy of how the muscles pull on the vertebrae. Each side is pulling equally, so the vertebrae stay in line. However, if one side pulls harder than the other, for example when one side is in spasm, the vertebrae moves in that direction. It is now said to be "out of alignment".

However, think about what will happen to the muscle if the bone is simply pushed back into alignment, without releasing the spasm that was pulling on it in the first place! The muscle will tear, or it will simply pull the bone back out of alignment again.

It is common, while I am working on a client's back, to hear the vertebrae "click" back into space as I release the tight muscle spasm – and take the strain off the vertebrae. If you should experience the "click" while you are self-treating the muscles of your back, you have just witnessed the result of the "tug of war" that the muscles play with the bones!

The back has a primary group of muscles with the fancy Latin name Erector Spinae, which means "erect spine." The Erector Spinae enables us to stand erect. There are several conditions that are adversely affected by spasms in the erector spinae group. First of all, these muscles originate on your rib cage. So, if there is a spasm in one of the fibers, that rib will not be able to move freely when you breathe. You will either feel a stabbing pain in the rib area, or you simply won't be able to take a nice deep breath.

Another back problem is caused by some muscle fibers, called "multifidi", which originate on the spine, connecting each vertebra to the one above & below it. These muscles are like little straps holding the vertebrae tightly together. When one of the multifidi has a spasm pulling on its insertion, it draws the two vertebrae together - "stepping" on the disc that is in the middle. Take a look at the drawing and this will make sense. We describe this to our clients as a hand pressing down on a jelly donut – the jelly will push out of the opposite side.

If the muscles are pulling down on both sides of a vertebra, then the disc is being compressed and will eventually herniate, or rupture. Treating the spasms that are pulling on the vertebre will release the tension on the bone and the pressure on the disks. Don't be surprised if you feel your vertebre "click" back into proper position, even though you aren't pressing on the bone. When the muscle spasms are relaxed the vertebre are no longer being pulled, and they return to proper alignment by themselves.

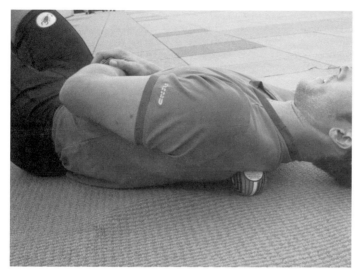

We will use a TP Massage Ball to self-treat this area. Lie back on the floor, bending your knees. Begin with the ball at the very top of your back, at the shoulder level. Stay on the ball for 30 seconds and then, by pushing your feet so your body moves up, maneuver the ball so it is rolling down toward the mid-back.

We are showing our athlete-model, John, with his body raised so you can see the position of the ball, however you need to be lying down flat to get the proper effect from the treatment.

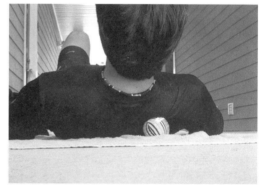

It's a bit tricky, but once you have tried it you'll see how easy it can be done, and practice makes perfect. You'll know exactly when you land on a spasm, you'll feel that "good hurt" we've been mentioning. If the muscle is seriously in spasm, it may be more than a good hurt, and you may have to ease into putting your full body pressure onto the ball. You'll know, when you find the spot, which way you should self-treat. Trust your intuition.

The Erector Spinae Stretch

This stretch is easy to do, however, it could take as little as 3 minutes, and as long as 30 minutes to be able to do it properly. The difference is how contracted the fibers are, and how often you do the stretch. It feels wonderful after you do it, so you know that it is worth the time

Sit cross-legged on the floor, with the entire length of your spine flat up against a wall. Make sure that you are pressing from your head to your tailbone (sacrum) against the wall.

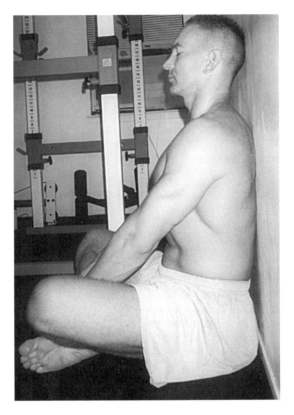

Next, the goal is to drop your head and have your chin touch your chest bone. The most important time to do this, and also the time it is the tightest, is in the morning when you wake up. If you take the time to do it, your entire day will be more comfortable. We tighten up a lot while we sleep and it could take hours to stretch sufficiently to relieve tension; this stretch greatly reduces that time.

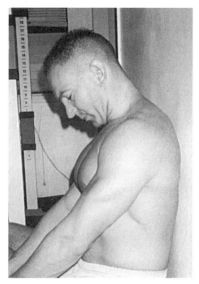

The trick is to bring your head down slowly, stopping as soon as you feel a bit of a stretch. Stay there for 10 seconds, and then continue to lower your head, stopping again when you feel the stretch. If you come to a point where you feel like a razor blade is cutting your back, just bring your head all the way up, move your head around, and then drop your head again. You will notice that the razor-like feeling has gone away.

Eventually you will have your chin on your chest bone. Now, stay there for one full minute. Again, if you have gone this far, and before the minute is up you feel the "razor pain", just lift your head up, move it around, and drop it again. You need to stay for 60 seconds WITHOUT pain.

If you have brought yourself to the point where it is very easy to do this on a regular basis (and that will come sooner than you imagine), now you can enhance the stretch.

After your chin has been on the chest bone for the minute. Continue to stretch your back muscles by keeping your chin to your chest and alternately raise each arm all the way up, really pulling up with your shoulder to extend the stretch to the latissimus dorsi muscle.

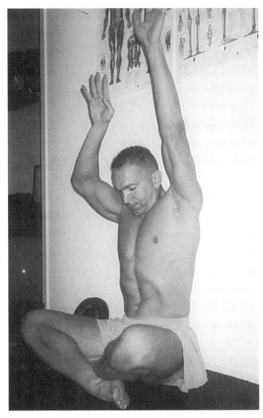

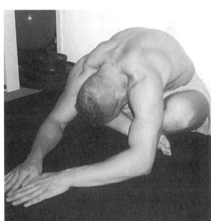

Picture #4 The next step is to begin to bend over, curling your shoulders in toward your chest and arching your back up, like a cat's. Bring your head down, as if you were trying to put your forehead into your lap. Alternate lifting one shoulder, then the other, drawing your arms forward.

You'll feel the stretch, and it will be wonderful. Do it slowly, enjoy the stretch. Spend at least one minute, more if possible, stretching your back.

You'll find that the more often you do this stretch, the shorter time it will take you to get completely loose.

132

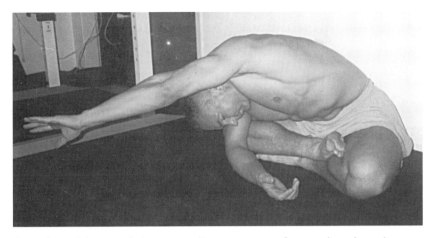

Complete this stretch by extending your arm forward and again reaching as far as possible to extend the stretch throughout the latissimus dorsi. This portion of the stretch can also be felt around the hips, stretching the lateral rotators, tensor fascia lata and gluteus muscles.

Along the entire length of the erector spinae there are many spasms that cause pain all over the entire back, and even into the chest and the hip areas. Also, around the middle of your back, right between your shoulder blades, are some muscles that cause pain in the same localized area. They are all treated by the next movement. Remember, none of these treatments should ever cross the line into intolerable. They should always be comfortable, even if they are a bit painful. If you are wincing for more than five seconds, you are going too far.

Add section from Runner's book that is on page 61 and 62, then continue the chapter as it is written in the Runner's book. Please note that the story and picture of Leon (pgs. 64-66) has been deleted from the Tri book.

The Iliopsoas:

The Foundation of the Body and Source of Multiple Problems!

It is amazing to learn that one muscle group, the Iliopsoas, commonly called the psoas (pronounced "so-as") can cause pain from the head to the toes. But it is absolutely true! We guarantee that most medical doctors, or therapists, will not consider your psoas muscle when you present to their office with joint pain or numbness anyplace in the body.

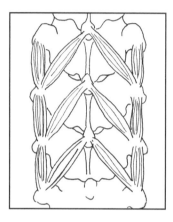

Before we examine the psoas, let's look at the logic behind the muscles that move the spine, and how the psoas causes such a wide area of pain.

Each vertebre of your spinal column sits on top of another vertebre. From your head to your sacrum, each vertebre is connected by small muscles called multifidi. As demonstrated in the graphic to the left, each multifidus muscle connects the vertebre on top to the one just below it.

There is also a long muscle called Erector Spinae that begins at the skull and ends at the sacrum area. While it appears to be one long muscle, it is actually thousands of individual fibers that originate on your ribs and insert onto the vertebre sometimes several levels higher or lower.

As each of these muscle fibers contract, the vertebre moves in that direction. It is an amazing system that allows us to bend our backs in the wide variety of movements that we take for granted – until something goes wrong!

The psoas muscle is the most incredible of these muscles because it connects the upper body to the lower body, and spasms anyplace along the length of the muscle will cause the vertebre of the low back to compress, and will also cause the vertebre of the upper/mid back to change alignment, referring pain into that area.

The Lower Back

Since there could be complicating issues, it is suggested that you visit your physician if you have been having severe pain in the lower back.

Pain in the low back is something that at least 70% of my clients complain about. And it is one of the most misunderstood conditions. As before, it easier if I use the proper names for the muscles. Please don't let the names scare you! They just describe where they are, and since all muscle names are in Latin, they look imposing. They aren't! The muscles are erector spinae, and the iliopsoas, which is called simply the psoas (pronounced "so-as"). It will help if you take a look at Chart 8 – psoas, and Chart 10 – erector spinae, while you are reading this explanation.

The erector spinae muscles are a large grouping of three separate muscles all closely placed together. Some originate on the ribs, others originate on the entire length of the spine, on each vertebra, and they all cause us to stand up from a bent position, or to be able to twist and turn our trunk.

The psoas originates on the lumbar (low back) vertebrae, it goes forward (behind your intestines), goes inside the bowl of your hips, and then inserts into the front of the femur – your thigh bone. The psoas muscle pulls you down, so you can touch the floor, and the erector spinae pull you back up to standing again. The psoas also is instrumental in you lifting your leg to take a step, or pedal a bike.

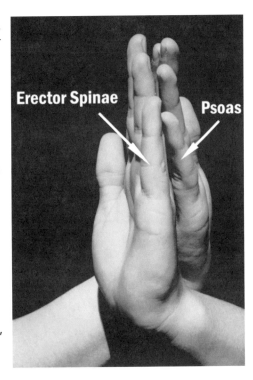

Let's spend a few minutes describing the location and action of each of these muscles. Cross your arms so your hands are back-to-back, with your fingers touching and pointing at the ceiling. Your left hand (which is now on your right) will be erector spinae, and your right hand (which is now on your left) will be psoas.

When you bend over to touch the floor the psoas contracts, and you are pulled over. Try it with your hands to demonstrate. Keep the back of the hands together and fold your right fingers down toward your palm. You can imagine the opposing muscle (erector spinae) needing to stretch to be able to do this move. When you stand back up straight, erector spinae contracts and psoas needs to relax. To demonstrate that movement pull the fingers of your left hand up straight, and have your right hand follow.

The problem comes from the fact that the psoas contracts many thousands of times every day, and unless we fold over backward, it never gets stretched! Both of these muscles originate on the lumbar vertebrae (low back), when either one of them goes into a spasm they pull on the vertebrae, and the pain is felt in the low back.

Since the erector spinae is stretching many thousands of times every day, it rarely goes into a spasm in the low back area – but it is common for the psoas to become contracted because of the phenomenon called "muscle memory". In this case, the muscle memory for the psoas is to be contracted! As the muscle contracts in a spasm it pulls the lumbar vertebrae forward and down, and you feel the pain in your low back! People automatically rub their back, but the pain is actually coming from the muscle that is located on front of the spine, and behind your intestines.

This is the reason why the pain actually feels a bit better when you bend over – you are going into the contraction and taking the pressure off the lumbar vertebrae. But, when you stand up, the muscle is again pulling on the vertebrae: pulling the bone out of alignment; compressing the disks; impinging on the nerves; and you are also feeling the tug of the muscle on the bone. The muscle definitely needs to be stretched!

Working with the athletes who come to our forum (www.julstro.com) has repeatedly proven another important factor of a psoas contraction - the fact that while the lumbar vertebre are being pulled forward and down, the pelvis is also being rotated forward.

This rotation causes a multitude of problems, including:

- Overstretched hamstrings which will cause pain to be felt at the top of the thigh/buttocks and also at the posterior knee. Since the fibers will be stretch so tightly, the hamstrings will appear to be contracted. You will either be treated for contracted hamstrings, or told you need to do hamstring stretches. However, you'll find that stretching the hamstrings only adds to the pain – a sure sign of a psoas contraction.

- Contracted quadriceps especially the fibers on the outside of the thigh. The quadriceps originate at the front of the pelvis, so as the pelvis is rotating down, the quads must shorten or they will be loose and unstable, unable to function. As they tighten to conform to the new required length you will lose strength. Also, the now shorter quadriceps will be putting pressure on the insertion point at the knee and you may feel pain when you try to bend your leg.

- All muscles that attach to the sacrum are pulled out of alignment. This will cause the piriformis muscle to press into the sciatic nerve and you may feel pain in your hip, hamstrings, calf, and the ball of your foot.

- The pelvis is pressing up on the sciatic nerve causing the same pain pattern as above.

- The femoral nerve, which exits the spine through the lumbar vertebre and then travels through the inside of the pelvis, can become entrapped and cause your thigh to become numb.

- The tensor fascia lata muscle of the hip is stretched and is therefore pulling on the ITB, and causing pressure on the lateral knee.

- The pressure on the knee often causes referred pain to be felt in the lower leg and ankle.

- The muscles that originate on the pubic bone are pulled back, causing groin pain.

- The entire vertebral column is being pulled from the bottom and causing disks to be compressed and nerves to be impinged along the spine – causing untold problems throughout your body!

It sounds incredible that one muscle can cause such havoc in the body, but we have seen this phenomenon in hundreds, if not thousands, of athletes and non-athletes. By simply releasing the tightness in the illiopsoas muscle the pelvis rotates back to its correct position and relief is felt in areas all over the body.

In fact, our experience has shown us that no matter what is happening to a person, do the psoas treatment and stretch before doing anything else. It's amazing how often this one treatment is all that is required to get a person back into a pain-free state.

As mentioned above, one of the quirks of a contracted psoas is the way it interacts with the quadriceps muscle group. As the pelvis is rotating forward due to the contraction of the psoas, it causes the quads to become shortened. If the quads didn't shorten they wouldn't have a strong base on which to pull. As a result, you now have a spasm, usually in the middle of the lateral quadriceps, that is also pulling the pelvis forward. A two-fold problem! In order to release the pelvis properly you need to alternate between the psoas treatment and stretch, and then the quadriceps treatment and stretch, and back to the psoas again. Continue going back and forth between the two areas until you feel relief of your back pain, or until you feel as though the two muscle groups are completely free of spasms and the fibers are fully stretched.

As we said at the beginning of this section, low back pain can be caused by other complicating factors that are more serious in nature than a simple spasm, but as long as you are cleared medically, we believe that the following treatment and stretch for the low back can also help you.

We had never been able to show a person how to successfully treat the psoas spasm until we discovered the TP Massage Ball. Cassidy, the developer of the TP Massage Ball, and the FootBaller, demonstrated his psoas technique and we're pleased to say, it works!

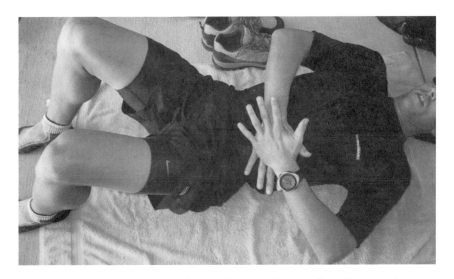

Lie on your back with your knees bent and your feet flat on the floor. Place the TP Massage Ball on your lateral abdominal area, just in front of your pelvis. Press the ball in toward your hip, with the intention on going to the INSIDE of your pelvis. You will be treating two muscles, the external oblique and the edge of the psoas muscle.

You are working in the area of the intestines and appendix, so it is important not to press directly down into your abdominal region, only press out toward the bone.

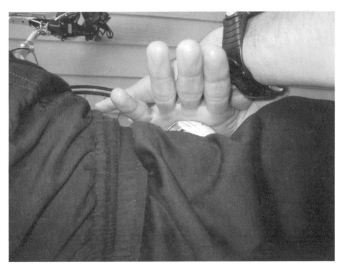

NOTE: To avoid putting deep pressure on vital organs you should only continue working the remainder of the abdominal area with your fingertips.

As mentioned, the (ilio)psoas never gets stretched. There are three ways of doing this effectively; you can use whatever way feels comfortable. Remember to only go to the point of a "feel good" stretch, not to the point of causing sharp pain. You will be able to go further each time you do it, and your back will feel better each time. As soon as you feel the stretch, slowly stand up straight. Don't hold yourself in the painful position. You'll be amazed at how quickly this helps low back pain!

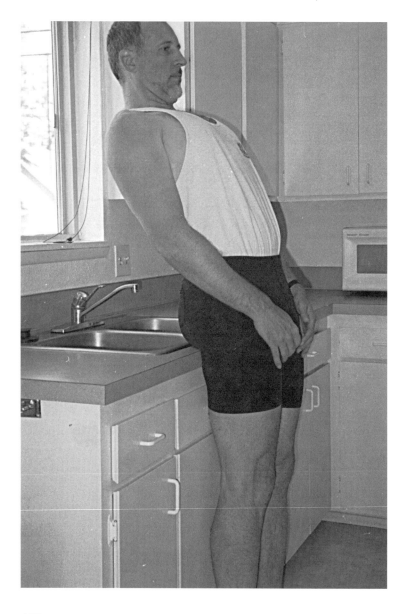

Turn around at the sink (see photo opposite page) – putting your calves up against the cabinet, and your hips resting against the counter. Keep your hips and calves touching the cabinet, also keep facing straight ahead, and lean back, moving your upper back over the sink. It helps if your lift up your chest, like you are trying to make a backward arch with your chest. This will raise the spine a bit before you lean back. Do this movement 10 times. On the last stretch bend forward, arching your back and moving your hips side to side.

Another method is done by lying on the floor on your stomach.

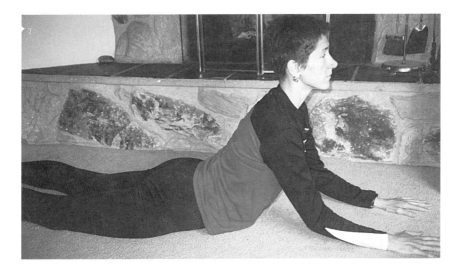

Do a modified push-up keeping your hips firmly on the floor, and bending backward at the waist. Go only until you feel a comfortable stretch, hold it for 6 seconds, and then come back flat onto the floor again.

Do this 10 times, trying to stretch a bit further each time.

On the last stretch, finish by folding at the hips and sitting on your feet. Stretch your back and put your head on the floor.

The third method of stretching the psoas is very interesting because it stretches both the psoas and the quadriceps at the same time! It was discovered by our friend Jerry Trump, when he was preparing for his first Ironman competition, and we're happy he shared it with us.

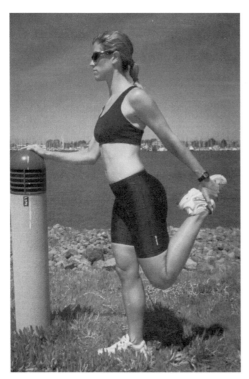

Stand up and hold onto a fence, or other solid object. Bring your ankle back and hold it with your hand, drawing your bent knee to a level that is behind the standing knee. After you have held this for approximately 30 seconds, bend your body back so you are actually arching your back and rounding your abdominal area. You will be stretching the psoas, and also stretching the quadriceps. Hold this stretch for another 30 seconds and repeat on your other side.

Finally, after you have stretched the psoas, it is important to treat the insertion point at the front of your thigh, and also to treat the quadriceps muscle (see – The Upper Leg). We have never had a client with psoas contractions who didn't also have a big spasm in the lateral (outside) portion of their quadriceps muscle.

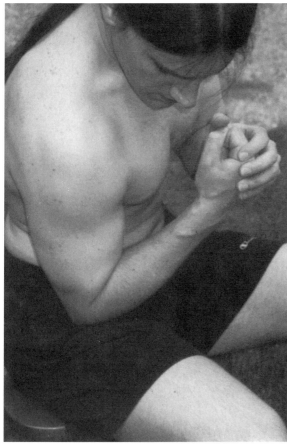

Sit down and find the crease where your hip meets your leg. Then go to the center of the crease.

Put your elbow directly onto the crease. Add pressure by pressing down with your shoulder. You'll know when you are near the spot. Hold the pressure for 60 seconds without pain. Continue doing the treatment until you feel the pain lessening.

You want to feel the pressure deep into the muscle and hip joint, while still staying in the tolerable range.

To stretch this area go to the section on quadriceps.

This is one of the "dual purpose treatments". As you are treating the insertion point of the psoas, you are also treating the origination of the quadriceps – and relieving pain in the anterior portion of your hip! This is a good time to continue the treatment and go down the entire quadriceps muscle.

The Quadratus Lumborum

The Quadratus Lumborum, "QL" for short, is the muscle that most people rub when they have low back pain. However, in our clinical practice we've found that it isn't the primary cause of low back pain - the psoas holds that distinction.

The action of the QL is to pull you over to the side, and it also picks up your hip so you can make a step – or sit down. Every time you pick up your foot the QL is contracting to allow that movement, and every time you sit down it is contracting to enable you to bend your leg. You can see how it can easily become overworked.

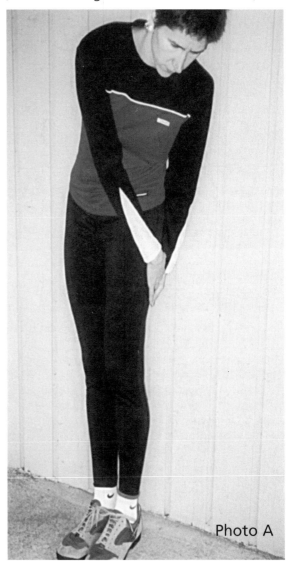

Notice that the referred pain for the QL, shown on TP Chart 11, is the same as that for the psoas. This is because, when you are sitting for a long period of time, or you have been running, walking or climbing stairs, the muscle has contracted. Then you try to stand up straight, but the muscle is too short for you to do that, so it pulls the lumbar vertebrae out sideways. This puts severe pressure on the spinal cord at the lumbar region, and you have low back pain!

Photo A

Any sport that requires a great deal of running: soccer players; football and basketball players; tennis; and naturally, runners, have a propensity for spasms in the QL muscle. Because of the location of the pain, you rub your low back. However, the muscle is underneath the very strong muscle of the back – the Erector Spinae. To effectively treat this muscle you need to stretch the fibers fully.

The stretch for the QL muscle is very effective, and one that has you looking like a pretzel.

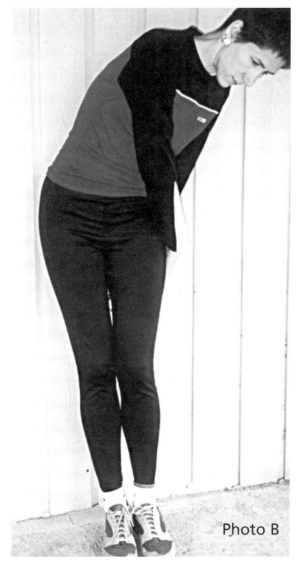

Photo B

Put your hand on your low back, at the curve of your waist, you'll be right on the QL (Photo A). Since the muscle goes up and down between the last of your ribs and your hips, the only way to stretch it is to move those two points apart. By adding a little bit of a twist to the movement, you get a better stretch than by just bending over to the side (Photo B).

Stand up with your butt pressed up against a wall. For demonstration purposes we'll stretch the left side, so you'll be bending to the right.

Keeping your butt on the wall, lean over to the right and then twist to try to touch your left hand to the back of your right leg. You won't be able to do it; in fact, you won't even be able to get close to the back of your leg. Just try to go as far as you can without moving your butt away from the wall.

Move your body about until you find the best stretch in your low back. Naturally, do this same stretch on the opposite side, even if you aren't having any pain in that area. The body compensates when we are in pain and we frequently will be straining the opposite muscle.

Again, be sure to keep this stretch at the "feels good" level.

CHAPTER 14

The Abdominal Muscles
The Core of Your Strength!

The four abdominal muscles form a girdle that expands from the top of the ribcage down to the pubic bone, and from one side of the anterior trunk all the way across to the opposite side.

The criss-crossing of the fibers gives support and protection to the ribcage and all the internal organs. The action of the abdominals is to flex the vertebral column and to compress the abdominal organs. Strong abdominals give you power in all your activities and help to protect your back from injury.

Weight lifters, in particular, cause spasms to develop in the four abdominal muscles, with the trigger points referring pain not only to the abdominal region, but also to the groin and low back! See Chart 7 to view all the areas affected by spasms in the abdominal muscles. In the case of the external oblique muscle, the spasms are located at the same points as the iliopsoas (psoas). The psoas is very deep and is not easily self-treated other than by stretching, however, the external oblique is a surface muscle and can be treated comfortably from a seated position.

You will be amazed at the number of spasms you will find, and you will be pleased at the result of the treatments. Spasms in the abdominals not only shorten the fibers, causing pain in the abdominal area; they also negatively effect the spine – causing back pain.

While looking at Chart 7, find the points on your body.

Use the opposite side hand to treat each point (left hand treats right side, etc.). Add strength to your treating hand by placing your same side hand on top of the treating hand. Simply find the painful spasm and press into it. Hold the press for 60 seconds, then move on to find other trigger points or spasms.

Weight lifters will have multiple spasms throughout the entire abdominal region, more than are shown on the charts. Just keep pressing into the muscle with your fingertips and you will know when you have hit a spasm! Treat each individual spasm as above

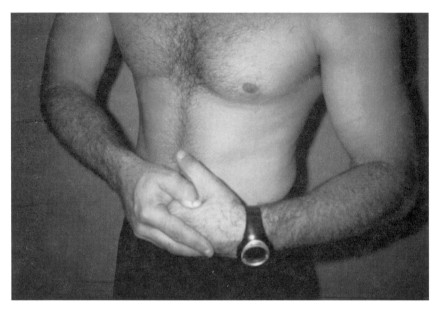

until you feel you have located each point. Chapter 13 showed how to do a treatment for the external obliques (lateral abdominal muscle) while also treating the psoas muscle.

While you are working on your abdominal muscles you will also find spasms in the intercostals that attach to each rib, causing the ribcage to open and contract during respiration.

Spasms develop in the intercostals muscles when a person is rapidly deep breathing – whether from strenuous exercise, or from coughing deeply. When you breathe in, the muscles must fully stretch to allow the lungs to fill. As the muscles contract, air is forced out of the lungs, and you exhale. It is clear to see that a spasm in these tiny muscles will prevent you from taking a deep breath – creating a lack of oxygen in your blood and also causing sharp "pin-like" pains in your chest.

Since the muscles run along the entire length of the ribs, you will need to press deeply between each rib to find any spasms in the muscles. Begin under your arm and deeply slide toward the center of your chest.

As with the abdominals, use your opposite side hand to find and treat the spasms. Use the same side hand to add strength to the movement. Treatment is the same as with the abdominals.

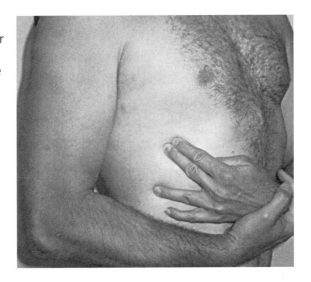

To stretch the intercostals, simply take a long, slow, deep breath. Don't hold your breath at the end of the inhalation, instead, slowly breath out as far as possible. Do this 2-3 times.

The Serratus Anterior and the Sternalis Muscles

While not an abdominal muscle, the serratus anterior muscle (see Chart 8), and the sternalis, (see Chart 6) are treated exactly the same as the intercostals shown in the above picture. The serratus anterior muscle is the cause of pain in the chest and down the arm, and of pain that is frequently thought to be caused by muscles of the back. The sternalis causes pain to be felt in the center of the chest and around the front of the shoulder.

It is important to treat these forgotten muscles. Your blood needs all the oxygen it can possibly get when you are competing, and spasms in either the abdominals or intercostals muscles will inhibit your ability to breathe deeply.

CHAPTER 15

The Many Faces of Hip Pain

The hip is second only to the shoulder in the amount of flexibility that it allows, and yet we pay little attention to its mobility…until something goes wrong!

Our hips swivel in an amazing number of angles, each movement being directed by a separate set of muscles all working in unison. Remember, muscles are like a pulley system. For any movement to happen, one set of muscles must contract, while the opposing set of muscles must relax. As a result, the potential for any one of those muscles going into spasm, and altering the function of all the other muscles, is enormous!

Athletes have a disproportionate amount of hip pain because of the frequency and duration of exercise periods. Many sports such as: cycling, running, bodybuilding, tennis and golf, etc., place an enormous amount of stress on the hip muscles. The fact that these are all done repetitively in the exact same direction causes specific muscles to spasm, with common areas of pain developing for each sport.

Fortunately the muscles are all close together, so treating one muscle usually benefits several other muscles. We will be addressing the major muscles in each area, but you are actually working on many muscles with each treatment.

This chapter and the shoulder chapter compete as potentially the longest in the book – there are so many spasms that cause hip & shoulder pain. You will be using a tennis ball frequently for the deep muscle treatments. Roll onto the ball slowly, and always stop before the pain passes your tolerance level. With that in mind, let's begin with the #1 cause of hip pain: piriformis syndrome, which often causes the pain of sciatica.

Sciatica – A Real Pain in the Butt!

The interesting thing about sciatica pain (if there can be an interesting thing about pain!) is that you cannot find a position that relieves the pain, and yet a simple stretch can alleviate it totally.

The sciatic nerve is actually the continuation of the spinal cord. When the cord reaches the sacrum (the flat bone at the base of your spine) it splits in two. Each division is now called the sciatic nerve. The sciatic nerve travels through an opening in the pelvis, and down the back of the leg. The complicating factor here is that the piriformis muscle originates at exactly the same point where the sciatic nerve exits the pelvis, through an area called the Greater Sciatic Notch. When the muscle goes into a spasm it presses the sciatic nerve into the bone - causing the symptoms of sciatica.

The piriformis muscle is frequently overlooked completely, and yet when one thinks of the anatomical placement of the muscle and nerve, it is the first thing that should be addressed when evaluating sciatica.

Actually, a better name for the pain you are experiencing is Piriformis Syndrome.

Charlie Chaplin's famous walk is an example of severe piriformis contraction. People who are most prone to piriformis syndrome are: runners, people who climb many stairs or work out on a stair climbing machine, individuals who sit for many hours at a time (including in a car or at a desk), and men who keep their wallets in their back pockets.

Several years ago we had a client who had an extreme case of Piriformis Syndrome. Jan was only 27 years old when she developed hip pain. The pain kept her up at night, and was with her all day. Her doctor ordered x-rays, and an MRI. Everything came back negative.

Eventually she was sent for physical therapy, but to no avail. The pain continued to get worse. After several YEARS of pain she was referred to a psychiatrist, who told her it was "all in her head" and put her on Prozac. Meanwhile, all of her friends were having fun, skiing, dancing, meeting men, and getting married – Jan was almost crippled from the pain and could not go out. She was depressed, and ate candy, not carrots. Needless to say, she gained lots of weight. This not only lowered her self-esteem, it increased her pain. Complicating her life further was the fact that she was in a dead-end job because it allowed her unlimited sick time.

When we first met Jan, she had been suffering for seven years. She walked with a cane and was bent over at the waist. Jan walked on her right toes because she could no longer straighten her leg. Her head was arched up to compensate for the bend in her back. Ironically, she came to the Julstro Center for shoulder pain. When asked why she was walking the way she was, she told us her story.

We thought, "With all the professionals who have seen this lady in the past seven years, it can't be just Piriformis Syndrome. Surely, one of them would have looked at the piriformis." Yet, Jan told us that no one had ever touched the muscle, they just gave her exercises, or pain medications.

Simply touching her piriformis muscle caused her to scream. It was so contracted that it felt like a bone! I began working with her, very gently at first, in order to bring some blood into the area, and soften the muscle.

After the first hour's treatment, Jan stood up. She was still bent over, and still stood on her toe. When I asked her if she was in pain, she said "no", so I told her to slowly put her foot on the floor – stopping when she felt pain. Miraculously, she was able to put her foot down flat on the floor. Then I told her to slowly stand up. Jan looked like a scared rabbit, and when she got all the way up straight, we both cried and hugged.

It took three months of frequent treatments, but one day Jan said "Julie, I can honestly say I have no pain in any part of my body!" We were thrilled. Unbelievably, her insurance wouldn't pay for deep muscle treatment, even though it paid for years of physical therapy, several MRI's, a psychiatrist, lots of Prozac, and many orthopedist appointments. Amazing!! This was one of the motivating factors for the development of the Julstro self-treatment system.

The location of the piriformis muscle is right under the hip pocket of your pants.

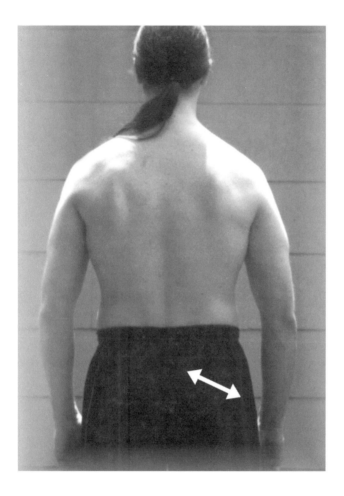

The piriformis originates on the sacrum (the big triangular bone at the base of your spine) and goes over to the hip (called the greater trocanter). The action of the piriformis is to turn your foot out.

The best way to self-treat the piriformis is to begin by using a soft ball, such as a child's ball, and work up to deeper treatments where you will use a TP Massage Ball.

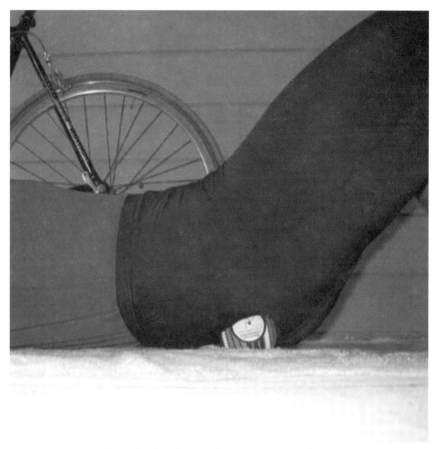

Position yourself so the ball is at the piriformis which is approximately in the middle of your buttock area and GENTLY roll onto the ball.

Lie on your back on the floor. If you are unable to lie on the floor, use a firm mattress. Have your knees bent and your feet flat on the floor. By altering your body pressure keep within your pain tolerance level. Stay there for 30 seconds and then roll your body further onto the ball. Do this until you are completely on the ball and you are feeling no pain. Then stay there for one full minute. If you feel pain during that minute, move off a bit, take a breath, and begin again. You should be able to stay comfortably resting on the ball for one full minute.

Several years ago I had a personal bout with sciatica pain that ended up having me learn the best stretch I've ever encountered for the piriformis. I was told to do it every hour for several days, and while that may sound like a lot, it takes time for a muscle memory to change, and the muscle to attain a new, longer set point. This wonderful stretch has worked for me, and it's worked for many of our clients. It's easy to do, and the results are amazing!

The Piriformis Stretch

Stretching the piriformis muscle is the most beneficial treatment you can do to either prevent, or heal, the pain of sciatica. It's an easy stretch that is quick acting, if you do it properly, and frequently.

The key here is the placement of your knee as you move your leg. I think it's best to read this treatment and look at the pictures, then print out this page so you can look at the pictures again while you're actually doing the stretch.

Lie on your back, on the floor if possible, and bend both of your knees. You'll have the best results if you do this to both legs, even though you are only feeling the discomfort on one side of your body.

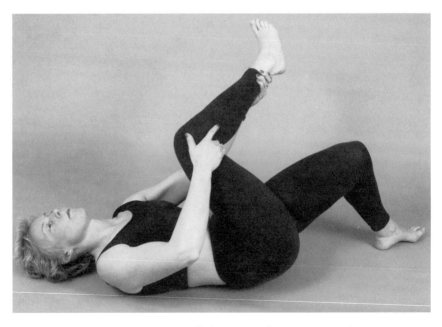

For demonstration purposes I'll show you how to stretch out your right muscle.

Bring your right knee to at least the middle of your body, having your knee in line with your nose. If you are flexible enough you can go further to the left, but you need to be at least at the midline.

If you find this position difficult, then this is your first goal to achieve. Once you have your knee at least at midline, hold it there with your right hand.

Next, put your left hand under your right ankle, and pull your right ankle up toward your left shoulder. Obviously you can't actually bring it there, just move it horizontally in that direction. Your level of flexibility will direct you regarding how far you can move.

Throughout this entire stretch, keep your back and shoulders flat on the floor.

For those less flexible, have someone help you with the stretch. Lie down, and while your assistant supports the weight of your leg with one hand, he/she guides your knee into midline. Once there, the assistant can begin to gently turn your leg to get the maximum stretch for the piriformis muscle.

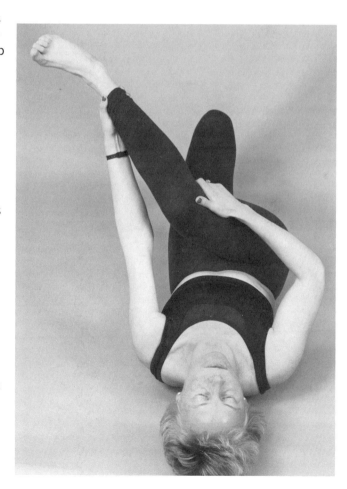

You'll feel a nice stretch in the buttock – the piriformis muscle. Keep the stretch at a level where it feels good – if it feels "sharp" back off a bit. The stretch needs to be held for one full minute. When the muscle feels like it's easing up, simply move your right foot more toward the left shoulder. Muscles need to be retrained to stay lengthened after they have been contracted for an extended length of time. The more times you do this stretch throughout the day, the faster the pain of sciatica will disappear. When we have a client who has a private office, we tell him/her to do it every hour! It works 95% of the time.

The Gluteus Minimus –
The Second Most Common Source of Hip Pain

> *"After running hard, for over 2 hours, I had severe pain in my knee. I've already had personal experience using the Julstro techniques to heal several serious conditions, so I've come to know not to rub the area, but to look for the source of the pain. The pain was so severe I could barely walk, but the chart showed the spasm was in my hip, in the gluteus minimus, even though I didn't have any hip pain. When I pressed on the point that was shown in the chart, a searing pain shot down to my knee! I did the Julstro technique, alternating with the stretch, for 15 minutes. When I finished the pain was completely gone! I'm back to training at my optimal level, and I've added another preventative self-treatment to my routine."* Jerry Trump

The gluteus minimus muscle and the tensor fascia lata are both responsible for pain in the knee, and for hip pain. The gluteus minimus also mimics the pain of sciatica. Look at Chart 14 and Chart 17 to see the referred pain areas from these two muscles; they cover a large percentage of your hip and leg!

The tensor fascia lata (TFL) muscle is right where your fists would go if you were putting them on your hips. The gluteus minimus muscle is at a point that is between the tensor fascia lata and the piriformis. The action of this muscle is to pull your leg directly out from the body. As a result, this is a muscle that is frequently strained in kickboxing, soccer, & wrestling, although it is a common area of pain for many people. The gluteus minimus is a major source of pain mimicking the same symptoms as the piriformis, and like the piriformis, the best self-treatment is with a tennis ball.

To find the proper place, stand up and feel your hips. Find the bone that is just below your waist, and then a few inches below it is the bone of your leg. The fleshy part in the middle is the gluteus minimus. Just below this spot is the tensor fascia lata muscle commonly called TFL.

Because the TFL muscle goes into a tendon that stretches all the way down to your knee, it refers pain to your knee. Most people don't think of their hips when the pain is at the knee!

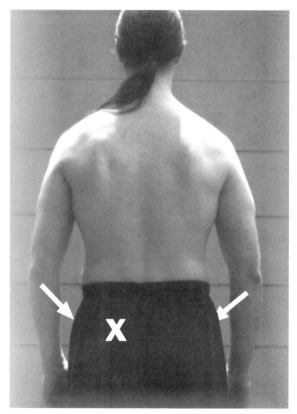

The location of the piriformis is shown with an "x" (only shown on one side of the body). The tensor fascia lata is shown with arrows. The gluteus minimis is between the piriformis and the tensor fascia lata.

Working in this area, and moving the TP Massage Ball just a little by just turning your body slightly, will get each of the muscles at the same time – it's one of the bonus treatments!

These muscles not only cause hip pain, but pain down the back of your leg (TP Charts 13, 14, and 17). You can alleviate lots of problems by working in this one area.

Now that you've found all of the muscles, lie down on your side. In order to treat the tensor fascia lata, put the TP Massage Ball right at the fleshy part of the hip, and roll GENTLY onto the ball.

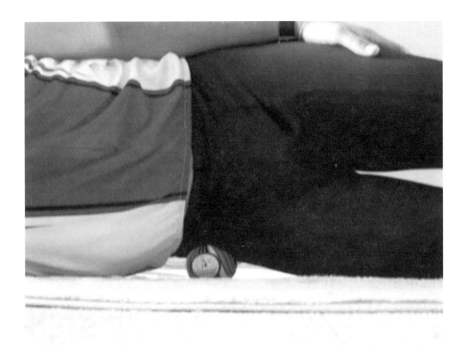

As always, stop if the pain starts moving toward intolerable. Hold each point for 60 seconds.

You will know instinctually when you are on the trigger point. It will be tender, and you'll know that you've found the problem.

After you work the TFL muscle, roll over a little onto your back.

You'll now be on the gluteus minimus, gluteus maximus, and gluteus medius in the back. Plus, with just a little movement you can reach the insertion point of the quadratus Lumborum by placing the ball on the top of your posterior pelvis.

The gluteus muscles are just about where your pant back pocket begins, and very close to the piriformis.

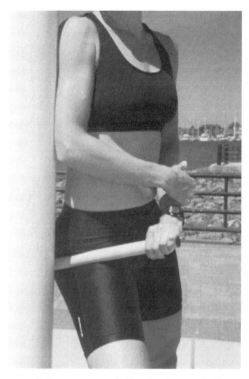

Another treatment that works very well on the tensor fascia lata was developed by an elite athlete with severe hip pain. This is a powerful treatment for the TFL so go gently and increase pressure as you feel necessary. Secure a dowel between your hip and the corner of a wall, of if your outside, use a tree or a fence to hold the dowel in place.

Position the dowel so it is on your TFL and then lean your body into it, rotating your body to get all the muscle fibers of the hip. You can finish this treatment by taking the dowel and working your quadriceps, especially the lateral fibers so you are also working on the ITB.

The following stretch for the TFL is for people who are flexible – and have good range-of-motion in their hips.

To demonstrate treatment on the left side of your body, put your left leg across the front of your right leg. Bring your left arm up and over your head, and bend toward the right side.

To get the full benefit, move your hips about a bit, until you feel the stretch. You should feel it about 3 inches back from your hipbone, and along your left posterior ribcage.

You can alter this stretch by moving your raised arm in different directions. This will give an additional stretch to the latissimus dorsi (Lats).

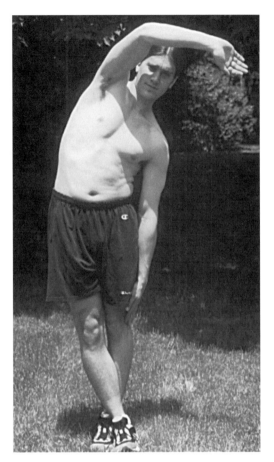

Insertion Point of the Psoas – A Source of Hip & Low Back Pain

Another place that causes low back pain, and anterior hip pain, is the point where the psoas muscle and the quadriceps meet. This point is directly at the top, and a little toward the outside, of the thigh. When you work on the quadriceps muscles (see - The Upper Leg), you will also be treating this source of the pain, however, the insertion point of the psoas is easy to treat by using your elbow.

While seated, find the crease where your abdomen meets your leg. Then go to the center of the crease. It's a bit tricky, but if you press around with your elbow, you'll locate it.

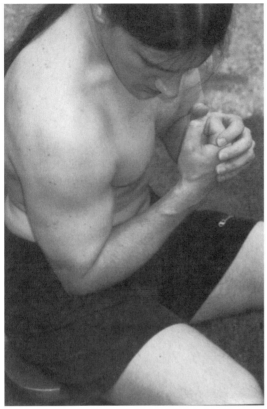

With your elbow on the crease, add pressure by pressing down with your shoulder and moving your elbow slightly toward your knee. You'll know when you are near the spot.

The idea is to hold the pressure for 60 seconds without pain.

Work with the pictures; they will help you do the treatments correctly. These treatments have been instrumental to many people in relieving their chronic hip pain; we hope they will be of benefit to you.

The quadriceps also cause pain in your hip. Each treatment assists in releasing the other muscle contraction. As a result, it will help if you combine this treatment with the treatment for the quadriceps.

However, we've found the quads usually affect the knee, more than the hip, so we've put the description of how to work them in the chapter for the upper leg.

CHAPTER 16

The Upper Leg – Knee and Hip Pain!

Working with Ironman Triathletes has been incredibly rewarding, and has demonstrated how important it is to work on the muscles of the quadriceps (called "quads" for short), the hamstrings in the thigh, as well as the gastrocneimus ("gastroc") in the calf. These muscles are a major cause of knee pain – for very logical reasons, once you understand the logic of the body.

Knee pain is a common complaint among all athletes. For example, cycling keeps the knees bent for extended periods of time, which will contract the hamstrings; and the forceful movement of pushing down on the pedals causes the quadriceps muscles to powerfully contract. Both of these muscles cross over the knee joint, and when the muscle is shortened from a contraction, it places enormous strain on the knee. Each muscle will pull on the knee joint, moving the bones out of alignment.

When a client comes in with knee pain, the first place we check are the quadriceps muscles.

Quadriceps – The front of the thigh – and Knee Pain

Because they originate on the front of the pelvic bone, when the quads are tight they throw the pelvis out of alignment. Think about what would happen if your pants were attached to the front of your hips, and you pulled down hard on them – you'd feel the pressure in your hips.

Likewise, if your pants were attached to just below your knee and you pulled up hard, you'd feel the pressure on your knee.

The quads are a major source of hip and knee pain for many people. The result of contracted quads, including a very common spasm that occurs midway down your thigh, either directly in the center, or just to the outside of the centerline (see TP Chart 17) is that your knee is being pulled toward the tight muscle. Frequently this is thought to be a ligament problem, however by simply releasing the spasms and stretching the fibers of the quad muscles you can totally relieve the knee pain.

Several years ago a client showed us how vital the "quads" are in relieving knee pain. She worked on a computer all day, and played tennis in her free time. She complained about her back and shoulders regularly, but never spoke about her knees. One day she said she was going in for knee surgery, and that she would be missing her next week's appointment. She was upset because she didn't think she'd be able to play tennis for two months.

I checked the quads since tight muscles would complicate recovery. On examination there was a huge spasm right in the middle of her thigh. It was 3 inches by 4 inches in size.

Releasing her quads was initially very painful, but as the contraction went down it became more tolerable, and eventually did not hurt at all.

We were surprised when she came in the next week for her regular appointment; we had expected her to be recuperating from the operation. She told us that when she went home after her appointment, her knee felt fine. Then the next day, her knee still felt fine. Since her knee pain had <u>completely</u> disappeared she canceled the surgery!

The second client was even more dramatic. Leon came in to the office after having had unsuccessful surgery on his low back. We were both surprised when working out the psoas muscle in his back relieved his back pain, making him realize that all he had as a tight psoas and that he hadn't needed surgery at all. He mentioned that he was also having severe pain in his left thigh and hip. Leon runs on a regular basis, is an avid tennis player, and was told he could never play again! The doctor told him that scar tissue from the surgery had wrapped around the nerve, and he needed additional surgery to remove the scar tissue. He absolutely refused, saying "I didn't need the first surgery; I'm not going for the second one!"

On examination, there was a huge spasm on his left thigh. Releasing the spasm had an immediate result. Leon got up from the chair and his pain had completely disappeared! Before explaining the treatment, let me finish by telling you that Leon has been able to go back to running and plays tennis every week. He's thrilled, and now that he knows how to treat his own leg and low back, he can be confident that the problem will not return.

If you look at the quadriceps, you will notice that the tendons of the quadriceps join together, and become the patella (kneecap) tendon. The tendon crosses directly over the kneecap and inserts on the bump just below the kneecap. Since the kneecap is a moveable bone, when a quad spasm pulls up on the tendon, the kneecap moves with it.

Depending on which of the four quadriceps muscles is doing the pulling, that is the direction that the kneecap will go, pulling the knee out of alignment.

The quadriceps treatments that work best to find the spasms and lengthen the fibers are:

Sit on the floor with your leg bent and hold the TP Massage Ball in your opposite hand. Press deeply into your inner quadriceps moving from the pubic area all the way down to just above your knee, do not use pressure as you return to the top of your leg. You will be treating not only the quadriceps, but the gracillis and the adductor muscles as well.

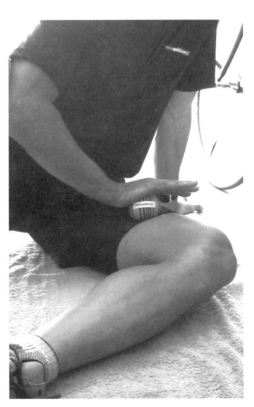

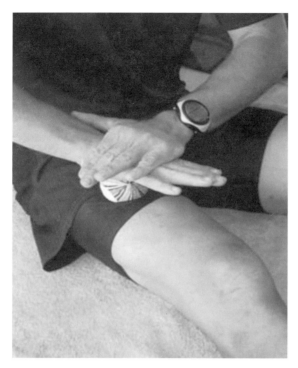

Deeply work out the spasms in the medial quads putting pressure only going down toward the knee.

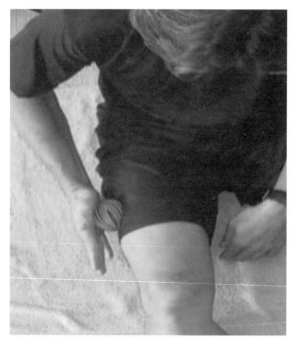

Then put the TP Massage Ball so it can roll down your lateral quadriceps and the ITB, again using pressure only on the movement toward the knee.

Finish the treatment by using a piece of 24" long, 2" thick dowel (i.e., a clothes closet pole) and while seated place the dowel at the very top of your thigh, where it meets your trunk. Press down and slide down the length of your thigh stopping just above your knee. Do this treatment to the inside, middle, and outside fibers of the quadriceps.

This treatment is more comfortable if you are wearing long pants.

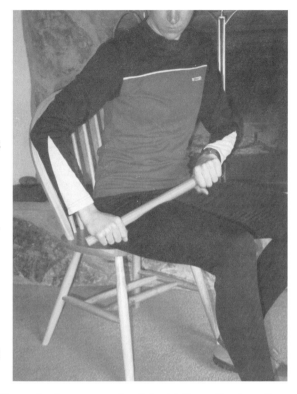

You can also use a rolling pin, however, don't hold it on the handles and let it roll, instead, hold it on the solid center, and slide it over the muscles.

The quads are big, thick muscles, so it will usually take several passes before you will begin to feel relief. If you find a particularly painful spot, just press down on it. The natural tendency for people is to avoid pain the moment they feel it, while just the opposite is what is necessary to relieve the spasm.

Do not go over the kneecap; stop about 2-3" before you reach that point. If you feel an area that is especially tender, you have found a spasm. Hold the pole on the spasm for a few moments, applying as much pressure as you can tolerate. Eventually this area will not be tender on subsequent treatments.

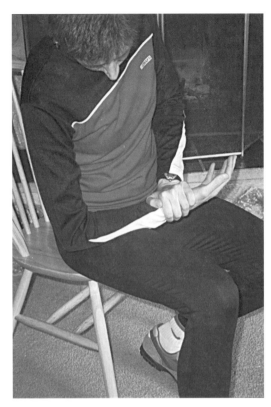

An alternative is to use your forearm. The bone, which goes from the elbow to the wrist, is your "rolling pin" (it's actually your ulnar bone).

To achieve the best results your thumb should be facing up. Lean in with your shoulder to put enough pressure on your quads. Simply push all the way down your thigh.

Do this several times, and always stay within your tolerance level. Remember, these are thick and deep muscles, so light pressure will not do.

As they say in the Marines "no pain – no gain", but with all of the Julstro treatments the pain must stay within your tolerance level.

The Quadriceps Stretch

The quads are very powerful muscles, and are also very difficult to stretch. Most people are familiar with the stretch that has you stand on one leg, taking the opposite ankle in hand, pull the leg back. This is effective to a degree. The two primary shortcomings are (1) some people can't balance on one leg, and (2) a stretch needs to be held for one minute. Also, if a spasm already exists, the stretch isn't effective in dissolving it. So, do the treatment described above, and then stretch the muscle.

The quadriceps are tricky muscles to stretch. If you kneel on the floor, sitting on your feet, you'll be in a good position to do an effective stretch.

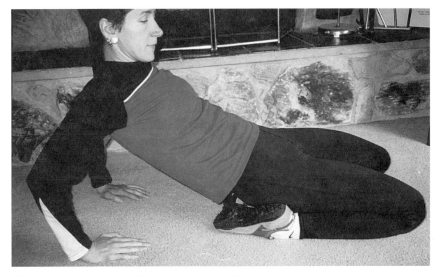

Simply lean your body back and you'll feel the stretch. Hold the stretch for 60 seconds.

If you are very flexible you can lean all the way back to achieve the maximum stretch.

This is a treatment that anyone who runs, climbs lots of stairs, or drives for long distances should do. Rarely do the muscles themselves hurt– they usually refer pain to other places. You'll be pleased when you see how this helps to make you feel more flexible in both the knee and hip area.

Hamstrings – The Back of the Thigh

In 2001, I decided to learn how to ski. While on vacation, I had a serious accident – completely severing the MC (medial collateral) Ligament on the inside of the knee, and slightly tearing my AC (anterior cruciate) Ligament, which is in the back of the knee. These ligaments are the strong fibers that hold the knee together. When any of the ligaments tear the knee loses some of its stability, depending upon which ligament is involved.

The muscles of my quadriceps and hamstrings had contracted into multiple spasms that tightened the, causing a great deal of pain, and instability, in my knee. My knee felt like it was going to collapse toward the inside, and I felt shaky walking, and going up and down stairs. I didn't think I'd ever be able to ski again – since even walking was "tricky".

Immediately after the accident I began self-treating what felt like hundreds of spasms in my quads and hamstrings. The pain was so severe that even touching my thigh hurt, but I knew it had to be done. As the pain began to lessen, I thought "how glad I am that I know these techniques" and was more determined than ever to teach them to others.

After Dr. Cohen examined my knee, and did an MRI, we decided to concentrate on strengthening the hamstrings in order to give support to the knee. To relieve the tension on the knee joint I would also self-treat all the spasms in the hamstrings and quadriceps.

Eventually I was able to increase my level of exercise, and also the level of self-treatment techniques to dissolve the spasms and stretch the muscles. Surgery was avoided, and my knee is back to normal. This experience was the catalyst for the self-treatments for both the quads and the hamstrings. Again, finding the answer on myself has been the most successful way to knowing how to teach others.

I went back to skiing in 2002, and skied my best ever! I was thrilled! My knee was completely healed by using the Julstro Techniques.

A very effective way to work out the hamstrings is to use a ball and work down three lines, following the muscle from the top to the bottom. For an especially tight, or tender, muscle use a soft ball on a soft chair.

To get more pressure, you can use a tennis ball, or baseball, on a hard surface. Look at TP Charts 13 & 14 for the referred pain areas of the hamstrings.

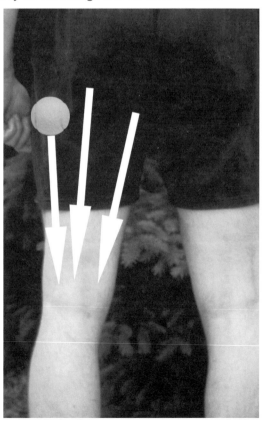

Begin by putting the ball at the very top of your leg. Make 3 lines down the back of your thigh. Begin all the way up at the crease in your thigh, where your buttocks meet your hamstrings, and work down each line to just above your knee. Sit down on the chair, putting your weight onto the ball, and hold it for 30 seconds before moving to the next point. You are looking for that "good hurt" here, don't overdo it.

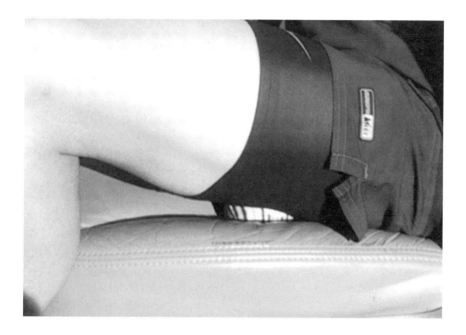

CAUTION: DO NOT press the ball into the back of your knee!

Finish off this treatment by stretching the hamstrings, and quads.

The Hamstrings Stretch

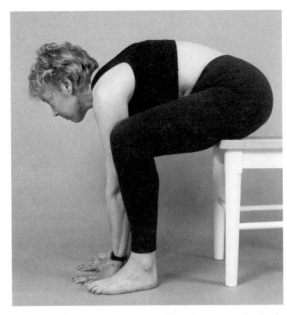

The hamstrings are tight on almost everyone we work on, especially athletes, and people who sit for hours at a time. For those of you who are physically able, the best hamstring stretch looks awkward, but works great.

Sit on the edge of a chair with your feet spread shoulder width apart. Bend over and put your hands FLAT on the floor between your feet. Keep your head bent up toward the ceiling as far as possible to prevent dizziness. Then – stand up!

Sounds easy – until you try it. You'll quickly find out how contracted your hamstrings are when you do this stretch!

Here's the key. As the muscle fibers stretch you can keep pushing your knees a little further back. Every 15-30 seconds lift your butt a bit more by pushing your knees back, and

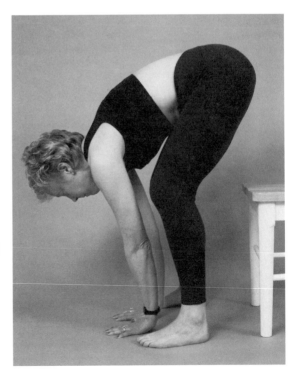

therefore stretching the hamstrings. Keep it up until you either straighten your legs completely, or you decide to sit down and take a rest. Try to continue this stretch until you are straight legged.

If the muscle is "burning", keep your hands on the floor, sit down for 10 seconds, and then stand up again. You will be surprised at how much further your legs will straighten.

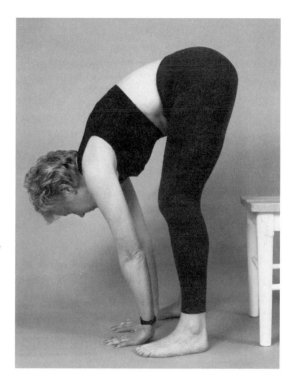

The beauty of this stretch is since you are starting with bent knees you cannot hyper-extend the joint, the position of your back is better for your spine, and the chair is right there should you get dizzy. You'll be pleased when you see how much better your legs will feel.

Another contributing factor to many people with knee pain is a muscle all the way up in the hip. The Latin name is Tensor Fascia Lata, and is called "TFL" for short. The chapter on hips gives you the method to work out the spasms in this area.

A method of stretching the hamstrings that is also safe for your knee is to lie down on the ground and put a long length of rope under one of your feet. Bend your opposite leg to take the pressure off your low back, and then lift the leg you will be stretching.

Keep your leg straight and pull up on the rope, so your leg is not doing the lifting but is instead being raised by your arms pulling on the rope. Go as far as comfortable, then stay there for 15 seconds and then again draw the rope tighter to move your leg up more.

Keep doing this stretch and hold action for at least 60 seconds.

Groin Pull

The searing pain of a groin pull can stop an athlete short. The most common muscle to cause a groin pull is the gracilis muscle. This muscle originates on the pubic bone, crosses the back of the knee joint, and inserts into the inside border of the tibia (lower leg). When this muscle contracts it assists in bending your knee, it also rotates your knee inward, as a result, pain can be felt in the groin, or in the knee.

To feel the muscle contracting, sit in a chair, place your fingers on the inside of your thigh, at the top of your leg near the pubic bone, and then pull your knees together. You will feel the origination of the muscle contract. If you kick your foot out while you are running, you are straining the contracted gracilis muscle. You are also straining it when you work with abductor equipment at the gym. To balance the muscles of the inner and outer thigh, it is important to treat spasms in the gracilis, as well as spasms in the quadriceps, sartorius and tensor fascia lata.

When the muscle is contracted, and shortened by spasms, it pulls on either the knee joint or the pubic bone. As a result, this muscle refers pain to the groin and is often responsible for male athletes having pain in the prostrate area, and female athletes having pain in the ovarian area. Your doctor may do a complete work up for this, ALWAYS take the tests, but while you are waiting for the results, do the following treatment.

Sports such as running and biking are particularly hard on this muscle because they involve bending the knees. This pulls the muscle to its longest length. However, if the muscle is shortened by a spasm you will feel the tension at the groin or the knee.

The treatment is easy. Get a 24" length of clothes pole (like in your clothes closet) and sit at the edge of a chair. Place the pole as far up on the top of your inside thigh as possible, and GENTLY press down toward your knee.

This can be very painful, so go slowly.

The majority of the spasms will be found closer to the top of the inside thigh, but may go all the way down to just before the knee joint. As you self-treat, don't press into the pubic bone. You can take your fingers and gently press on the two insertion points at the pubic bone and the inside knee.

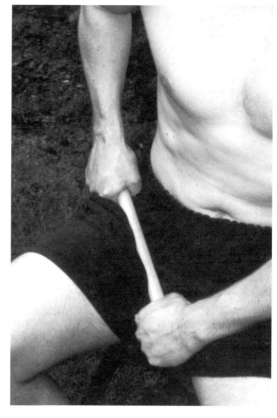

We suggest you put ice on the muscle after you work it out; also, arnica gel is great for bruised muscles. Apply it frequently over the entire area.

The Back of the Knee

The forum on our website (www.julstro.com) demonstrates how common it is for athletes to have posterior knee pain. Behind your knee is an important muscle that causes athletes to suffer with so much pain that it can make it impossible to extend the leg from a bent position. The muscle, called popliteus, originates on the front of your knee on your femur (thigh bone) and wraps around to the back of your knee on the posterior side of your tibia going about 3" below the bend at the back of your knee. The anatomical attachments of this muscle are important to note because it explains its nickname "the key that unlocks the knee".

When the popliteus contracts normally it causes the knee joint to open by bringing your lower leg up toward your hamstrings, "unlocking the knee" so the more powerful hamstrings can continue to raise your lower leg. When you straighten your leg the popliteus must stretch to its longest length. However, if the popliteus is in spasm it can't stretch, but you are forcing your leg to go straight, and the muscle pulls on the insertion point on the back of the knee. The tension causes you to have a burning pain focused directly behind your knee.

Another muscle, called the plantaris, is also located behind the knee and also causes pain to be felt when your leg is straight. The plantaris muscle originates on the back of the femur, crosses over the knee joint and inserts into the Achilles tendon. When it contracts it assists your knee in bending, and when it is in a spasm it causes pain in both posterior knee and the ball of your foot, occasionally going all the way to the big toe!

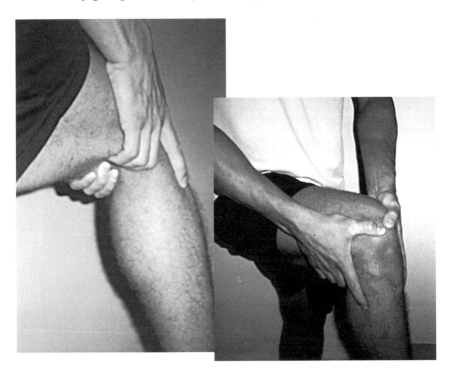

One treatment will quickly eliminate the spasms in both of these muscles. Bend your knee and wrap your hands around your knee joint. Have your middle fingers directly into the area behind your knee joint and your thumbs on your knee cap. You are using your thumbs as leverage and pressing into the muscles with your middle fingers. Move around an inch in any direction until you find the tender point and then maintain the pressure for at least 60 seconds. End the treatment by slowly straightening your leg while you are still maintaining the pressure on the muscle. Do this two or three times, or until you feel relief from pain.

"It is amazing to me that we can treat ourselves!"

I first met Julie Donnelly at Ironman USA in Lake Placid. At the time I had a chronic ankle sprain and iliotibial band irritation from a previous marathon. She showed me in 10 minutes how to self treat my injuries. I was so impressed with my relief from the pain and the return to normal function that I subsequently signed up for her newsletter and have been consistently using her treatment system to treat any of my tight/overused muscles.

Annalisa

Age group triathlete, equestrian, and distance runner from Quebec Canada

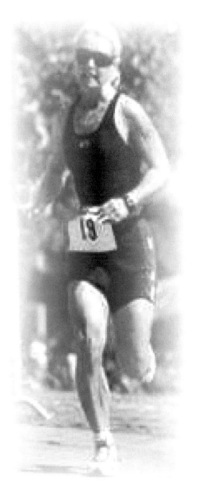

CHAPTER 17

The Lower Leg

> WARNING: Many conditions require medical attention from a qualified physician. "Bumps" in the tissue of the lower leg in particular, can be signs of a serious medical condition. Swelling of the lower limps can also be symptoms of serious conditions as well. Never apply pressure to varicose veins. Always see your doctor before using the Julstro techniques.

The Nemesis of Many... The Source of Ankle and Foot Pain...and Shin Splints!

Shin Splints

A common complaint from athletes who do a lot of running in their sport: soccer, tennis, basketball, football, baseball, as well as running and jogging, is shin splints. Deep, burning, pain radiates down the entire front of the lower leg, often from the knee to the ankle. The pain can eventually become so severe that you can't point your toes, and even slow walking is extremely painful.

The problem comes from a severely contracted tibialis anterior muscle. Look at the tibialis anterior muscle and you will see that it is a long thick muscle that runs along the entire length of the shinbone, and its tendon inserts into the top outer portion of the foot.

When the muscle of the shin is in spasm you can feel the pain either as shin splints, or as pain in the outside/top ankle, depending on the degree of the contraction and the exact location of the spasm. Look at TP Chart 15 to see the referred area of pain. Notice that the pain goes all the way to the toes.

If you run your finger directly down the muscle, while at the same time bringing the front of your foot up off the floor, you will feel the muscle contracting. Follow the muscle all the way over the front of your ankle, just a bit toward the inside, and you will feel the tendon as it tightens. The muscle then goes across the top of your foot, under the arch and inserts on the bottom of your foot. As a result this muscle can also cause pain in the arch.

Since the muscle contracts every time you lift up the front of your foot, every step you take contracts the muscle. If you run, and don't finish off each step by pointing your toes, you are contracting it far more than you are stretching it. Ultimately muscle memory sets in, and it shortens. As we have discussed throughout this book, when that happens the muscle pulls on the tendon and you feel pain at the insertion.

Many people experience pain from this muscle, for example those who do a lot of walking or driving. Runners are especially prone to experiencing pain at both the origination along the shinbone

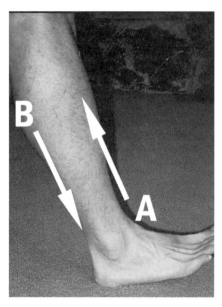

because the muscle is actually pulling along the length of the bone; the top of the foot where it bends at the ankle; and the bottom of the foot because of the insertion of this muscle. When the tibialis anterior is contracted you frequently get a burning type of pain, or it feels like you banged it very hard and have a deep bruise. Each time you push off from a step, you point your toes down and pull the heel up. If you are feeling pain on the inside top of your foot, it is because the muscle is tight, or shortened, and now you are stretching it slightly with every step you take.

You must flush out the spasms, lengthen the contracted fibers, bring fresh blood into the area, and stretch!

Walk a little and watch the action of your foot. As you take a step you point your toes up, contracting the tibialis anterior (A) and stretching the calf muscles (B).

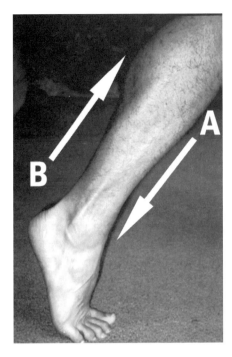

Then as you push off from your toes, you are stretching the tibialis anterior (A) and contracting the calf muscles (B).

When any of the muscles are shortened the pulling will hurt at the insertion point. The fact that the tendon goes under a band at the ankle, and that the tight tendons rub on the band, is the reason why this muscle can cause pain on the top of the foot close to the ankle.

The treatment is the same for both shin splints and ankle pain, so we'll discuss both here. Shin splints are a common condition for any sport in which running is an important component, especially if it is sustained running for any period of time. The tibialis anterior muscle contracts so strongly that it actually begins to pull away from the bone!

This treatment is easy, but it can be quite painful. We recommend warming the area before you do any deep therapy. You can warm it by taking a hot bath, using moist heat compresses, or prior to exercising you can use the heel of your opposite foot and quickly rub up and down the muscle.

The Julstro self-treatment for this condition is to lie down on the bed or floor. Have your lower leg exposed, or you may be more comfortable wearing tight pants, and remove your socks.

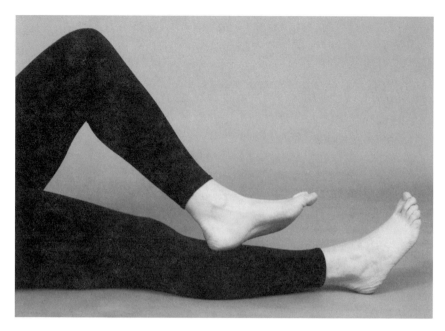

Demonstrated on the right leg: Take the heel of your left foot and place it just to the outside of the shinbone, all the way up near the knee. Now, apply pressure by pressing down on your left heel and DEEPLY slide down the right leg, and over the ankle. Press your heel all the way to the top of your foot.

If you feel any pain at any point you have found a spasm in the muscle. STOP and put sustained pressure on the point. Do this several (8-10) times, trying to increase the pressure with each pass.

As you are pressing down onto the muscle, stretch it toward the direction of your foot. As you lengthen the muscle fibers you are relieving the tension from the tendons, you are also drawing fresh blood into the muscle, and you are pressing the fibers back down onto the bone.

Since this can be a tender area, only use enough pressure to work the muscle, but still be tolerable. The chances are that you will not get this muscle to be pain-free after just one treatment, although the pain in the ankle should lessen with the first treatment. Do it for several days in a row.

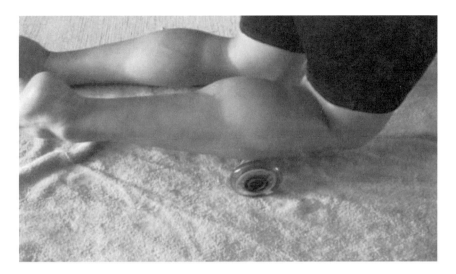

A very effective treatment for a tight tibialis anterior muscle is to use the FootBaller. Place your shin into the crossbar of the FootBaller and slightly turn your leg so you are not resting on your shinbone, but are instead resting on the top of the tibialis anterior muscle. Move your leg so the FootBaller rolls down toward your ankle, keeping the pressure deep, but tolerable.

You can also use the TP Massage Ball to work on the tibialis anterior muscle. Again, start at the top of the muscle and then move your leg so the ball rolls down toward your ankle.

This can be a painful treatment so start with gentle pressure and work deeper as the pain begins to subside.

Immediately next to the tibialis anterior is a muscle called the Extensor Digitorum Longus. This muscle travels down the outside of your leg along with the peroneal muscles. They insert on the top of your foot and on the outside of the foot. Together they lift your foot and angle it so pressure falls onto your big toe. TP Chart 15 demonstrates the pain pattern for the Tibialis Anterior, and for the Extensor Digitorum Longus.

Pain in the ankle can be caused by the peroneal muscles; TP Chart 17 demonstrates that pain pattern.

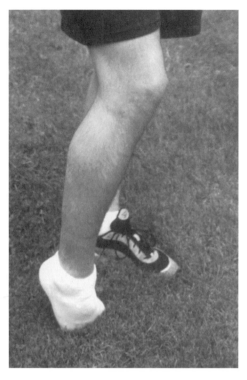

The way to stretch the tibialis anterior and the peroneal muscles is to point your toes down as far as you can while turning your foot so the toenails, and the length of your toes, are pressing into the ground. Put pressure onto your toes until you feel the stretch of the muscle.

Another way to stretch the muscles is bending by your knees and sitting on your lower leg while your toes are pointed.

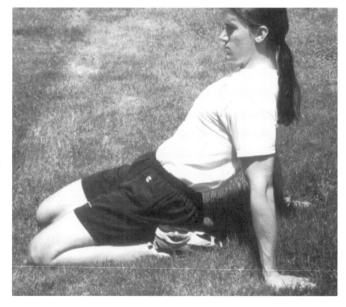

Many athletes have pain along the inside of the tibia bone, just opposite from the tibialis anterior muscle, and it can refer all the way to the ankle. The culprit is the origination of the soleus muscle and it can easily treated by taking the heel of your opposite foot and pressing into the bone at exactly the point of the pain and directing your pressure down toward your ankle.

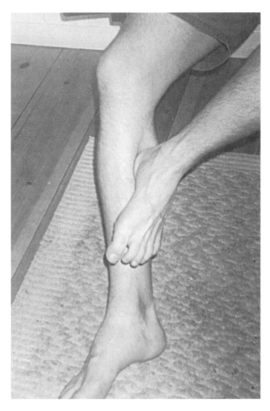

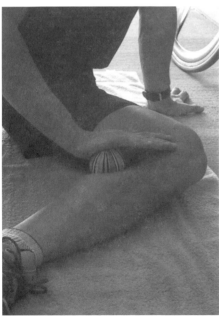

Another alternative method of treatment is to take the TP Massage Ball in the opposite hand and put it at the top of the inside border of your tibia bone. Press down deeply and roll the ball toward your ankle. If you find an especially tender point stay on it for 30 seconds and then continue the movement. Do this several times.

The Calf and Achilles Tendonitis

Jerry is a Triathlete. His goal for the last several years has been to compete in an Ironman distance event. He worked towards it for years, and it was finally in sight. Then he developed Achilles Tendonitis. After a year and a half of trying every remedy doctors had suggested, he was barely able to run three miles before the tendonitis would force him to stop. There was no possible way he was going to be able to train enough to compete.

Have your legs ever gotten so tired that they throbbed? Do you get cramps in your calf? Have you been diagnosed as having "Achilles Tendonitis"? Have you ever had a heel spur? Often these are the natural responses of the body to contracted muscle fibers in the calf muscles.

Runners have a propensity to Achilles Tendonitis. This is the condition that occurs when the two muscles of the calf are pulling so tightly onto the tendon that they are actually trying to tear the tendon off the bone!

As the muscles shorten, the tendon pulls, and you lift your heel. However, as the muscle goes into a shortened state, and stays there while you are putting your foot down flat on the ground, the tendon is being pulled so severely that it can either tear away from the bone, rupture the tendon, or cause a heel spur. This last condition, heel spurs, happen because the muscle is trying to tear the tendon from the heel, and the body sends bone cells to hold onto the tendon. This keeps going, the muscle pulling and the body sending bone cells, until a spur developes.

An inflammation at the insertion point of the Achilles tendon is the first step toward potentially tearing the Achilles tendon. Medications may relieve this pain, or may simply take away the inflammatory response, but they only mask the symptoms while ignoring the cause. It is vital to release the spasms in the two calf muscles: the gastrocneimus (gastroc for short) and the soleus!

We have often had people complaining about pain in the Achilles tendon area even when the muscles leading to the AT (gastrocneimus and soleus) are both found to be without spasms. There are two muscles that lie just under the AT, called flexor digitorum longus (inserting on the bottom of your toes) and flexor hallucis longus (inserting on your big toe. These muscles pull the foot back during a step, and are contracted totally when a person is running. As a result, any sport that involves running will likely cause these muscles to go into a spasm. When they shorten they put pressure on the heel and by referral, to the entire bottom of the foot.

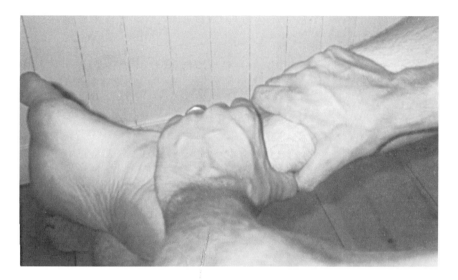

The treatment for the muscles is to put direct pressure onto the area on either side of the AT. You can do this by pressing deeply with your thumbs, or

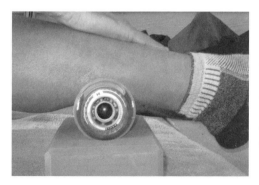

by placing the posterior ankle area onto the FootBaller and moving your leg so the pressure is applied from the point where the soleus and gastrocneimus merge into the Achilles tendon, all the way to the heel bone.

Heel Striker Pain

Another condition that is often found in athletes is extreme tenderness on the bottom of the heel, and possibly along the inside, and outside, border of the foot. It is possible that the bone is bruised from hitting the ground, with great force, with each step. A bone bruise can take a long time to heal. However, contractions in the gastroc and soleus can also cause pain to radiate through the heel and the foot. The treatment is the same as for Achilles tendonitis. The result may be slower than the Achilles tendonitis treatment, but it will help ease it immediately, and with frequent treatments, the pain will eventually disappear.

As you look at the muscle chart for the gastroc and the soleus, notice how they merge into the tendon. To release the tension on the spasm you will need to treat the calf muscles.

We have noticed that most people have seen, or used, the stretch for the "gastroc" muscle - the top muscle of the calf - but they aren't aware that there are two muscles in the calf. Under the "gastroc" is a muscle that, while hidden from view, is just as important when addressing pain in the calf or heel. That muscle is called the soleus.

Take a look at TP Chart 14 and you can see the trigger points on the gastroc. The soleus is under the gastroc, and can't be clearly shown on these charts. Both of these muscles insert into the Achilles tendon, the thick band at the back of your ankle, and then go to the heel bone. When they contract, your heel is lifted off the floor, and you are standing on your toes. The difficulty arises because even those people who do stretch frequently ignore the soleus, only doing the stretch that works on the "gastroc"

Before going into the treatment for these two muscles, look at TP Chart 13 – piriformis, TP Chart 14, and TP Chart 17 – gluteus minimus. You'll notice that calf pain comes not only from the calf, but from muscles far from the calf, so if local treatment doesn't help, look for the spasm elsewhere.

Prior to treatment, warm the muscles whenever possible. Use a heating pad for 5 minutes, and do some gentle stretching by putting your leg out straight, bring your toes up toward your shinbone, then rotate your foot in a circular direction.

As you move along the muscle during the following treatments, if you find a painful "bump", that is the spasm that needs to be pressed out!

Because they are on top of each other, the treatment will melt spasms in both of the lower leg muscles. Begin very gently with these treatments, calves can be quite painful! If you're flexible it's

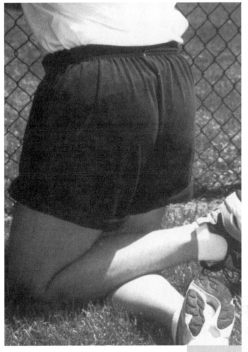

easy to do these treatments by using your shinbone as a rolling pin, so let's begin by demonstrating how to treat the right leg.

Kneel on the floor, holding onto a wall, or a chair. Use your shinbone to press down onto your calf.

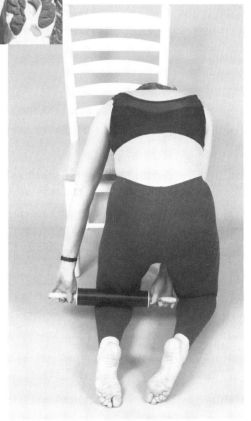

Alternatively, use an 18" length of dowel (or a rolling pin, in a pinch). Start up as close to your knee as you can get, DON'T PUSH BEHIND YOUR KNEE, and push it all the way down to your ankle. If you find any especially tender spots, stay on them for about one minute, and then continue down to the ankle. Do this several times on both legs.

You can easily treat both the gastrocneimus and soleus muscles by using the FootBaller placed on top of "The Block". Sit on the floor and place the FootBaller on top of the Block, then put your calf onto the crossbar. Move your leg so the FootBaller

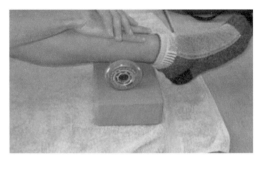

is pressing into your calf and it is rolling down toward your ankle. Use more pressure while going down toward your ankle than on the reverse in order to lengthen the muscle toward the insertion point.

You can cover the entire calf area by simply moving your foot so it is pointing in toward the midline, and then pointing out away from the body.

Because you run on a wide variety of surfaces, and in all kinds of weather, you can't always kneel down. This was brought to our attention while working with Jerry, the Ironman Triathlete previously mentioned. We needed to figure out a way that could be done in the cold, wet, weather in Washington State. He discovered how to do the treatment by balancing on a tree or road sign! Since Jerry discovered this technique, here he is demonstrating how to do it.

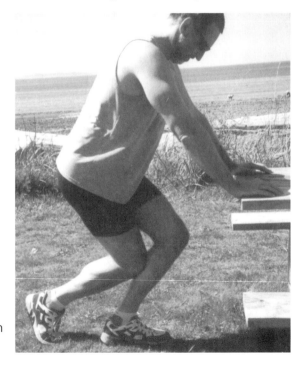

Hold on to a secure object, bend your knees and put your knee directly onto the calf of your sore leg. Hold this for 60 seconds, and deeply slide your knee down toward your ankle.

Do several passes down the calf in order to work the entire calf muscle.

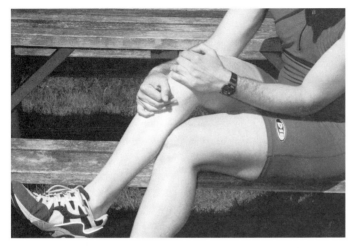

You can also effectively work on your calf muscles while you sit cross-legged in a chair. Simply put your calf directly on top of your knee - press down- and slide from the top of your calf to your ankle.

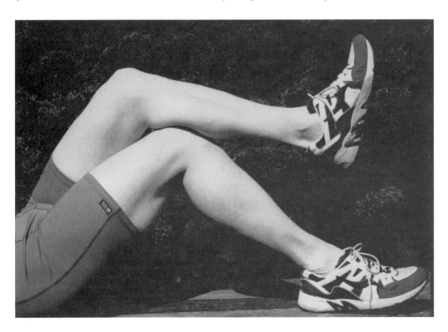

Finally, you can do this while you are relaxing! Simply put your calf on top of your bent knee and move your top leg to slide the kneecap under the calf muscle. Go from the top of the calf to the ankle.

Even if you are only feeling pain or tightness in one leg, do both legs. You'll be surprised how painful they both can be.

Muscle Cramps

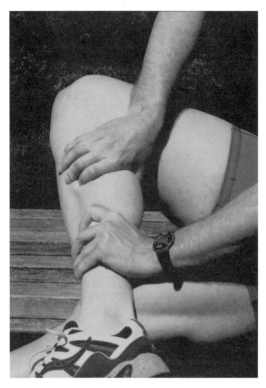

If you experience a sudden cramp, don't try to stretch out the fiber while the contraction is still happening. A muscle contraction will not stop in the middle of the pull; if you stretch it during the cramp you will be pulling it in the opposite direction and then you may tear the muscle fibers. This is one of the reasons that often a person will feel pain in the muscle long after the cramp has ended.

Instead of stretching and pulling on the muscle fibers, hasten the completion of the cramp by assisting the fibers in their contraction, and then stretch the muscle. The two most common places for muscle cramps are in the calf, and in the arch of the foot.

To hasten the end of a cramp in the calf muscle, tightly grip above and below the muscle – just below the knee and just above the ankle – and push your two hands together, shortening the muscle. This will be extremely painful for about 10 seconds – but the time will still be shorter than you normally experience when your leg cramps.

Hold the muscle together for about 15 seconds and then release. Repeat this same movement to help any last fibers to complete the contraction. The pain will be substantially less during the second movement.

Now you can move into the treatments for the calf muscles – the soleus and gastrocneimus shown in this chapter.

The arch of the foot is treated in a similar manner.
Grip your foot around the ball at the base of the toes, and at the heel. Then push the two ends together as much as possible. This treatment is fast, and less painful, because the muscle is so short.

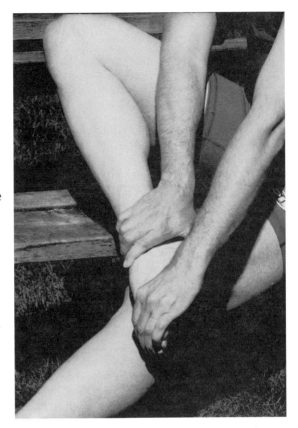

After treating the foot cramp you can proceed to stretch it out by standing up on your toes and leaning forward. You can also push your thumbs deeply along the arch - as if you were trying to lengthen the muscle from the heel toward the toes.

Finally, if your toes begin to cramp, sit down and using your fingers, press deeply in all the areas around the base of the toe, and in the areas in between each of the muscle tendons to the foot. Also, press into the ball of your foot, arch, and work up your leg. There will be places that are very painful – you'll know when you find a spasm. Just hold your finger pressure on it for about 60 seconds; you'll feel it melt away.

Lower Leg Stretches

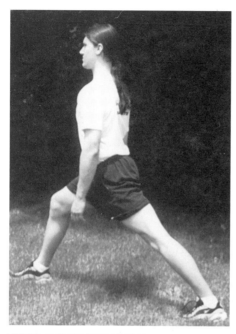

Most people know about the stretch for the gastroc. We teach it without bending forward to lean on a support, so you can do it any place easily. Look at the pictures as an example of good posture: keeping your back straight will be more comfortable.

To stretch the gastroc, put one leg forward, and the other back. Keeping your foot flat on the floor, bend the forward knee.

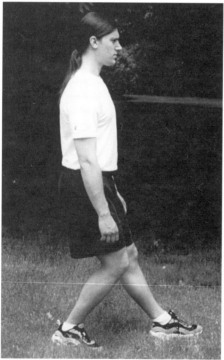

To stretch the soleus, stay in the same position as for the gastroc, then move your body back a bit and bend your back knee. You will feel the stretch in a totally different location.

We've had runners who are shocked at how different they feel when they stretch the two muscles, instead of just one. The relief felt is wonderful!

Finally, the last lower leg muscle we will work is the Peroneal muscle group.

Stand up and put your leg onto a chair, or sit on the floor or bed.

Roll your foot out toward your little toe and turn your leg so you can better reach the muscle. Using the length of dowel, press onto the outside border of your leg, just above the ankle. Lean back and slide the pole up your leg, stopping just below the bone of your knee joint.

If you find an area that is especially tender, that is the spasm. Using the dowel, press on it, try to flatten it, and stretch the fibers. These are forgotten muscles, and are rarely stretched, or flushed out by the majority of massage therapists. Yet, a little treatment goes a long way with the peroneals. Flush them out and your ankle will move easier, any nagging discomfort can be quickly relieved.

Next to the tibialis anterior is a muscle group called the peroneals. The peroneals are actually three separate muscles: peroneus longus originates at the top of the fibula (bone at the outside of your lower leg) and joins with peroneus brevis that originates approximately midway down the fibula. The tendons of both of these muscles go behind your heal and insert onto the side of your foot at the fifth tarsal bone (long bone between your heel and your toes). When in spasm these two muscles cause pain to be felt on the ankle bone.

The short muscle peroneus tertius originates on the lower part of the fibula, passes under the band at your ankle, and inserts at the same point as the other two peroneal muscle. The peroneus tertius causes the same burning ankle pain that is common for the tibialis anterior, and is sometimes mistaken as a symptom of shinsplints. The peroneus tertius also causes heel pain. When they contract normally you pull your foot out so your little toe is off the ground and the inside of your foot has rolled onto the ball of your foot. When the peroneals are in spasm they cause pain to radiate down the side of your leg and also causes sharp pain to be felt behind the ankle bone.

Runners are especially prone to having contracted peroneal muscles. Also, if you have ever sprained your ankle you will likely have a spasm in the peroneals and the tibias anterior muscles, potentially causing you problems for years until they are finally released. The reason is because as you twisted your ankle the muscles were overstretched, and then when you straightened your ankle they snapped back, but a spasm was created that will stay until it is physically released. We have seen people who have suffered with ankle pain for years after twisting their ankle, and yet just a few minutes of working on the spasms in the peroneals and tibialis anterior eliminates the pain immediately.

You can easily treat the peroneals with either the dowel or the TP Massage FootBaller.

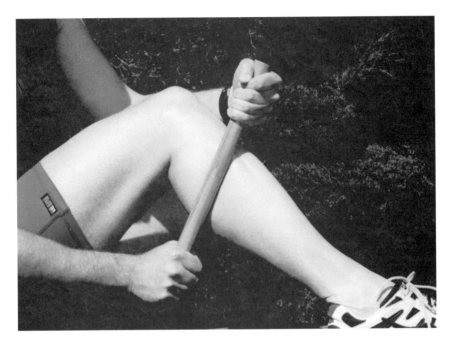

Stand up and put your leg onto a chair, or sit on the floor or bed.

Roll your foot out toward your little toe and turn your leg so you can better reach the muscle. Using the length of dowel, press onto the outside border of your leg, just above the ankle. Lean back and slide the pole up your leg, stopping just below the bone of your knee joint. If you find an area that is especially tender, that is the spasm. Using the dowel, press on it, try to flatten it, and stretch the fibers.

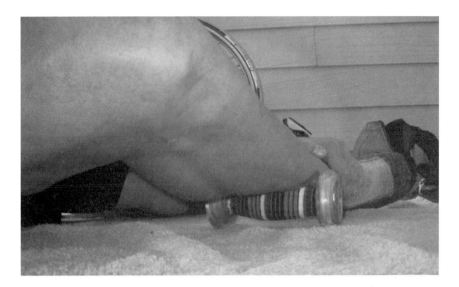

Another way of easily treating the peroneals is to sit on the ground and put the TP Massage FootBaller under the outside of your lower leg, just below your knee. Use your hands to press down on the inside of your knee and ankle, and move your leg so the wheel moves from just under your knee joint and stops just before you are pressing onto the bone.

These are forgotten muscles, and are rarely stretched, or flushed out by the majority of massage therapists. Yet, a little treatment goes a long way with the peroneals. Flush them out and your ankle will move easier, any nagging discomfort can be quickly relieved, and pains may disappear from as high up as your knee, and as far down your leg as your big toe!

CHAPTER 18

Foot Pain

All sports that involve landing hard on the foot, such as: running, tennis, soccer, basketball, and a wide assortment of other sports, can cause foot pain. Even swimming and cycling, sports that wouldn't be thought of as stressing the foot, cause cramping, and pain in the top of the foot.

Your feet are your foundation, when they are in pain you can't continue. We are sure you have already found the best footgear for your sport, and that you do the normal care for nails, arch support, and callous removal. We want to discuss how the muscles can cause pain and cramping – and how you can stop it short.

Many of the treatments for the foot are included in the Chapter 11 - The Lower Leg, because the muscles of the lower leg are responsible for the movement of the foot.

It has been our experience that the majority of people, when they feel pain in their foot, would not think to look at the leg as the source of the problem. However, the large majority of time, this is exactly where the problem is occurring.

Pain on the top of the foot, and pain in the arch, is often caused by the tibialis anterior and peroneal muscles on the front and outside of the lower leg. When you are running, you are contracting the tibialis anterior muscle in order to land on your heels, but you don't follow through with pointing your toes at the end of the step. One way to help relieve shin/ankle/foot pain <u>while you are running</u>, is to complete each step by pointing your toes as you push off.

Cycling keeps your ankle bent for hours, which means the tibialis anterior is held in a contracted state for hours. Eventually the muscle shortens (it's called muscle memory) and pulls on the tendon, causing pain at the top of the foot, as well as along the shinbone.

Heel pain and bone spurs are also frequently caused by tightness in the calf muscles. You will not eliminate these pains until you release the spasms in both the gastrocneimus and soleus muscles of the calf.

Plantar Fasciitis

Plantar Fasciitis means "inflammation of the fascia of the muscles on the sole of the foot". The foot has several important muscles that move the toes into various positions.

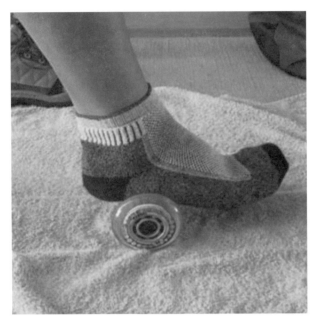

To treat the muscles of the arch and the sole of the foot, simply put the TP Massage FootBaller on the floor and roll your foot on it. Press it into the arch of your foot and roll it back and forth (from toes to heel & reverse). Go up into your toes, and along both sides of your foot.

There are two other important areas of the body that commonly refer pain to the arch. The first is the Piriformis muscle. This muscle is located under the back pocket of your pants. The muscle crosses over the sciatic nerve, and when it goes into a spasm, it presses the nerve into the bone (called the Greater Sciatic Notch), causing Sciatica. When the sciatic nerve is impinged, you feel pain in your hip, down the back of your leg, and into your arch. The Piriformis muscle is responsible for turning your foot out, which is a very common problem for runners.

The following picture demonstrates an easy way to stretch the piriformis when you have pain while you are exercising, and are you are unable to lie down:

Stand up with your leg out in front of you, your knee locked, and your foot pulled up.

Keep that position and turn your foot all the way into the midline - so your toes are pointing to the back of the opposite ankle. You will feel the stretch in your hip and buttocks.

This is a very important stretch for anyone who sits a lot, runs, or climbs stairs.

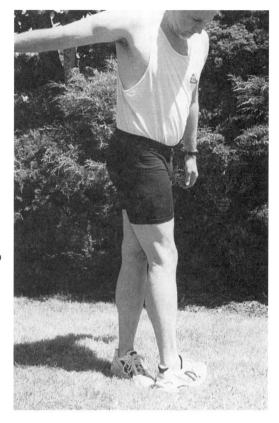

Another important area that causes plantar fasciitis, and Achilles tendonitis, is the muscles of your calf. A spasm here will try to pull the Achilles tendon away from its insertion at the heel, and will refer pain to the arch.

As demonstrated in Chapter 11 – The Lower Leg, the best way (there are several) to treat this is to sit down, cross your legs (sore leg on top) and press the center of your calf muscle directly into the knee of the opposite leg (see treatment in lower leg). Use your locked hands to add pressure on the top leg, pushing it further into the bottom legs kneecap. Make sure your foot/ankle is relaxed. Now, pull your top leg up, so the kneecap slides from the top of the calf down toward the ankle.

This treatment may be painful, especially as it passes over the spasm. Stay well within your tolerance level, this treatment may take several passes before the spasm begins to go down. Turn your top leg to try to treat the entire calf muscle.

Heel Pain (also see Chapter 11 – The Lower Leg)

Pain in the heel of the foot - on the bottom, inside border is also caused by the calf muscles. One would think of it as a "bone spur" in the pad of the heel, but in this case, it isn't. Work the calf muscles with your opposite knee, it is an important treatment when you have heel pain.

After releasing the calf muscles, use your fingers to deeply press down on the insertion point of the Achilles tendon, all the way down to the bottom of the heel. It takes a long time to really work this one out - but every time you do it you will have pain relief for a few hours. Gradually it getts better and better - hurting less and the treatment lasts for a longer time.

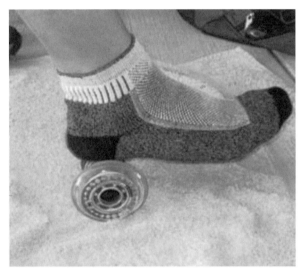

Finish the treatment by pressing your heel down onto the crossbar of the FootBaller, moving from the back of the heel all the way to the toes.

Sharp Pain in the Ball of your foot and cramping of the Toes

When this happens you may have spasms in the lumbrical muscles. These are small muscles that go between each of the tarsal bones in your feet, and up to the first joint in your toes. The tarsal bones are the long bones in your feet, that lead up to your toes.

Because of their insertion into other, longer, muscles, the action of the lumbricals is to assist in curling your toes up, and down.

As you are exercising, you are probably holding your toes one way, or the other, for long periods of time. Ultimately the muscles shorten (called muscle memory).

When they shorten, and you try to move your toes in the opposite direction, the muscle pulls on the insertion point. It feels like a sharp pin has been stuck into your foot - in between the toes, but down a bit toward the meaty part of the ball of your foot (base of your toes).

To treat them, take off your shoe. Cross your leg over so you can easily press into the ball of your foot, and also the top of your foot, between the tarsal bones. You'll just have room between the tendons, and the tarsal bones, for one fingertip. Press around, you'll find the spasms. It will feel like a tiny pea, or a tiny pebble.

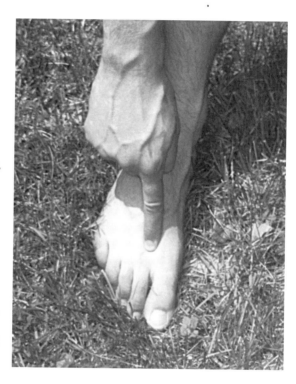

Press your fingers deeply into your foot, go in between all the tendons, between the bones, wherever you can find a painful point - that is a spasm.

When you find the spasm, hold pressure on it, as deep as is comfortable - and you'll feel it ease up. As it is getting less painful, the muscle spasm is melting. We suggest you keep poking around and look for any other spasms that may have developed in your feet.

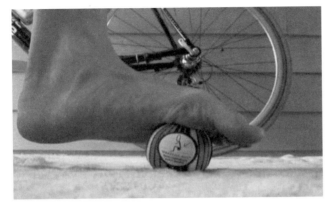

A TP Massage Ball is a wonderful thing to stand on and roll around under your toes, ball of the foot, arch, and heel. The FootBaller is another perfect object because it is smooth, it rolls, and it covers the entire bottom of the foot at the same time.

Spend time caring for your feet, without them you are completely "out of the race". A TP Massage Ball is a wonderful thin to stand on and roll around under your toes, the ball of your foot, arch and heel. The TP Massage FootBaller is another perfect object because it is smooth, it rolls, and it covers the entire bottom of the foot at the same time.

Your fingers, and these tools, will help you to find, and treat, many spasms. It's like a quick "foot reflexology" treatment. Your feet will feel great!

CHAPTER 19

Getting Race Ready

At the Start Line...or before your long training run

Congratulations! It's all come together and you are at the Start Line of the race. Your heart is pumping...your mind is rushing from place to place...you're warming up your muscles and trying to keep your thoughts calm by chatting with fellow runners. You only have 10 minutes to go and your body will be pushed to its limit – or beyond!

Take this time to prepare your muscles for the task ahead, focus your thoughts in a direction that will enhance your ability. It is important that you increase the circulation to each muscle group, and to assure that your joints are as flexible as possible. This is the pinnacle of your preparation and training. Use these minutes wisely!

As best as you can under the circumstances, try to find a space away from the hub of the action. If you can sit on the grass it would be ideal. To prepare your muscles and joints you will need just five minutes of concentrated efforts that will bring huge results.

Before you sit down, close your eyes, take in two or three slow deep breaths, visualizing oxygen filling your lungs completely and sending nutrients to each of your muscles. "Feel" a wave of relaxation flow down your body, from your head to your toes. "See" your muscles untying, lining up like elastic bands, well-tuned for the task before them. This 30-second meditation will actually cause your muscles to release tension that has been building as you moved toward the Start line.

- Begin your stretches with your neck (Page 104), and entire erector spinae of your back (Page 130).

- Loosen your shoulders by releasing any tension in your pecs minor (Page 108).

- Stretch your forearm muscles (Page 125).

- Stretch your psoas muscle (Page 140), doing the slow back and forth movement at least 5 times.

- Continue by doing one 30-second stretch for both sides of your quadratus lumborum (Page 144)

- Lie down in the grass (or if impossible, lean up against a tree or building) and bring one knee close to your body. Push it toward the opposite side and hold on to your ankle. Slowly move your lower leg up toward your shoulder and stretch your lateral rotator muscles, especially the piriformis. (Page 156)

- Lean over in a sitting position and placing your flat hands on the ground, slowly straighten your legs to stretch your hamstrings. Don't overdo it, just a nice gentle stretch. (Page 174)

- Sit down on the ground and using your forearm, push down on your quads, moving toward your knee. One or two passes is all that is necessary to flush out any lactic acid and bring in fresh blood (Page 167)

- Bend your knees and use the heel of your hand to push the lactic acid from your tibialis anterior muscle, stretching the fibers toward your ankle (Page 184).

- Gently push your knee down your calf muscles. Prior to a race you don't want to press too deeply onto this muscle. One pass on the inside-middle-outside is enough. This isn't a time to work out spasms so DO NOT be pressing in deeply. Your intention is to lengthen the fibers and draw blood into the muscle to nourish it as you run. (Page 192)

- If possible, find a big rock and step on it, rotating your feet to warm up the muscles of your arch and toes.

- Stand up and slowly rotate your entire body in every direction. Move your shoulders, your hips, your neck, in circular directions. All the while, visualize your muscles as strong, elastic bands.

Finish your 6 minute warm-up with another deep breath. Keep your thoughts on seeing yourself as you cross the finish line.

You are now ready to race – Good Luck!

While You Are Running

Your mind is all over the place. It goes from thinking of nothing, to watching the crowd, to thinking about aches and pains, and wondering if you are going to make it to the end.

It's amazing how the mind controls the physiology of the body, and it's important to focus your attention on what you DO want, keeping your thoughts away from what you DON'T want. If you allow your mind to focus on pain, it will intensify, so you need to be consciously aware when you find your thoughts taking you away from your goal.

When you are aware of pain, first think of what you can do to reverse it while you continue running. There are a few things that can help without causing you to lose time:

- If your shins or the top of your foot/ankle start to hurt, your tibialis anterior muscle is in spasm. You can stretch it while you run by exaggerating the movement of pointing your toes toward the back as you push-off from your step.

- Calf pain or Achilles tendonitis pain is caused by some or all of the muscles in your calf going into spasm. Exaggerate your step as you come down on your heel. This will give a slight stretch to the calf muscles

- Occasionally think to arch your back while you run. This will help to stretch the psoas muscle and will prevent, or alleviate, a whole list of possible pains.

- You are breathing deeply as you run, enhance the experience by visualizing oxygen as tiny pellets of nutrition being forced into your muscles.

- If you do stop for a water break, quickly flush down your quads with either the heel of your hand or with your arm. Use a pressure that feels good, you are trying to push out lactic acid that is building up from the muscle action. You will also be drawing in blood so it will help your recovery tomorrow.

- At the water break you can also wrap your hands around your thighs and quickly flush out your hamstrings, and then slide down to your lower leg and squeeze the lactic acid from the muscles of your calf (use your four fingers) and tibialis anterior (using your thumbs).

After The Race

You know the normal routine: drink lots of fluids, avoid chills, walk around to prevent muscles from tightening. You will heal much faster if you add a few things to your post-race routines

Use arnica gel as a lubricant and flush out your muscles from your hips to the arches of your feet. Simply squeeze &/or press your hands into all of your muscles. You are actually pushing the lactic acid out of the fibers. Your muscles are sore, so be gentle with your pressure, but vigorous in your actions.

Many athletes tell us they have success by taking arnica tablets before and after the race – 3 tablets every 15 minutes for two hours. This gets the arnica into the blood stream to heal the muscles from within.

Gently stretch each of the muscles. It is important to be gentle, your muscles are in an injured state, you need to nurture them.

If there is a massage tent, bring your arnica gel and ask the therapist to flush out your legs while using the gel. Ask them to press out the lateral rotator (hip) muscles and lightly stretch your back. Avoid any deep muscle treatments until two or three days after the race.

Get a good nights sleep – you deserve it!

A Few Other Thoughts

Arnica is a 200+ year old homeopathic remedy for muscle bruises. We have been told by many of the athletes who come into the office how taking three arnica tablets every 15 minutes for two hours prior to the race has greatly improved both the pain felt during the race, and also hastened the healing time after the race.

We recommend that you pack a tube of arnica gel into your waist pack for after the race. Generously rub it on your muscles, and keep rubbing it on frequently after the race.

Before you leave home on the day of the race, review the treatment for muscle cramps (Page ???). Hopefully you won't need it. Since stretching a cramping muscle can tear the fibers causing greater pain that can last for several days, it's important to have this technique in the front of your mind should you suddenly need it.

Finally....

Racing, and sports participation, is something that you can enjoy for your entire life.

Be sure to have your annual check-ups, eat properly, stretch, and get enough rest to compensate for the strain you are putting on your body.

If you treat your body right you will be rewarded with years of **"Pain-Free Living"**.

We wish you the very best as you grow in your sport. Please visit us at our forum on www.julstro.com.

"...after ONE treatment I resumed running pain free..."

This is the greatest forum I have ever been a part of! I had knee pain for weeks and after ONE treatment I resumed running pain free, and I have been running for two weeks pain free now. I am glad I did not wait seven months like I did with the shin splints. I tell every runner, or any person with pain for that matter, to check out your forums. The help and information you give out for free is a service that all people could benefit from, and the pain free runner was a priceless investment for me. Thank you so much for your time and your help.

Running pain free,

Mike

"For the first time in 2 weeks my legs feel almost normal."

I don't believe it! For the first time in 2 weeks my legs feel almost normal. Your treatments really work, thanks so much!! I hope it lasts. Considering I did a fairly intense running workout the last two nights, I believe that it will. Tonight is a rest night. Still doing treatments and stretching.

I'll be honest, I was afraid I had a stress fracture or a severely sprained ankle. I never thought that knotted up muscles could cause such discomfort.

My marathon is a week from Sunday.

Thanks, again!

Larry

"...this really worked!"

Just wanted to tell you that I ran the Olander Park 100 mile - and I FINISHED! I was the last of the under 24 hour people, but I'll take that any day. There were things happening to me that were new, and just because I had read your book, I was able to deal with them. I used my dowel numerous times, and the big one was a low shin pain that I remembered you said to point your toes after pushing off, and this really worked! I had to do it every so often for the entire race, but I wouldn't have known about it without you... thank you!

Ron

"After finding your website I felt like I had been set free..."

...the techniques I've learned from your website made it possible for me to complete my first half-ironman this past April. I've been doing tris the past three years being constantly plagued by one injury or the other. After finding your website I felt like I had been set free to really and finally enjoy this crazy sport. Thank-you so much for your invaluable service!

Angela

"This is going to be the one of the best books I have!"

I can't believe my abdominal cramps had anything to do with muscles in my legs!!! After many tests came out negative, I was losing hope I'd ever get rid of these cramps. I think this is going to be the one of the best books I have! I'm definitely going to spread the word about this.

D.D.
Massachusetts

PART IV – GLOSSARIES AND TRIGGER POINT / MUSCLE CHARTS

Appendix A - Glossaries

These glossaries are not meant as a medical dictionary. They are included for the convenience of the reader who has little knowledge about the body. Only those terms that are used in this book are included in the Glossary of Terms, and only the major muscles, and not all muscles discussed in the book are listed in the Glossary of Muscles

The explanations have been purposely written in non-technical language. For a more complete glossary, please check any good anatomy and physiology textbook.

Any muscle that was discussed in the text will be linked to a graphic of the muscle. Other muscles are included for your information even if they are not specifically taught in the Pain-Free series of e-Books.

Glossary of Terms:

Adhesion: When muscle fibers have an injury, they put out a substance that sticks the adjoining fibers to the injured fiber. This allows the injured fiber the opportunity to rest and heal.

Anterior: Toward the front of the body. (i.e.: your chin is anterior, your spine is posterior).

Arnica gel: A topical homeopathic remedy that heals bruised muscles.

Bone spur: A "bump" on a bone. A tight muscle that is attempting to pull its insertion away from the bone frequently causes a spur. The body sends the bone cells to hold the insertion in place.

Brachial Plexus: A group of nerves that originate in the neck and are responsible for the sensations felt in the arm, hand, and parts of the chest and back.

Breastbone: Common name for the sternum.

Carpal tunnel: Found in the wrist, it is an area that is formed by 8 small bones (carpal bones) as the base, and the flexor retinaculum as the bridge. Nine flexor tendons and the medial nerve pass through this area.

Carpal Tunnel Syndrome (CTS): A condition in which the median nerve is being damaged as it passes through the carpal tunnel.

Cervical Vertebrae: Neck bones.

Clavicle (Collarbone): The long bone located at the very top of the chest, it extends from the breastbone to the shoulder.

Collarbone: Common name for the clavicle.

Contraction (of a muscle): The natural movement of a muscle. When a muscle contracts (shortens), a joint moves.

Extensors: Any muscles that draw a limb away from its natural bend, i.e.; the extensors of hand straighten your fingers when they are bent, and the extensors of the leg straighten a bend of the knee.

Flexors: Any muscles that bend a limb; i.e., the flexors of the hand cause you to make a fist, and the flexors of the leg cause you to bend your knee.

Flexor retinaculum: The bridge of the carpal tunnel, the flexor retinaculum is the origin of several of the thumb muscles.

Frozen shoulder: A condition that is caused when many, or all, of the muscles that move the shoulder blade are contracted. The shoulder is unable to move.

Insertion (of a muscle): The area of a bone where the muscle ends. The muscle pulls this point, causing it to move toward the origination of the muscle, i.e., the hamstrings insert on the lower leg, so when they pull the knee bends.

Isometric exercise: A type of exercise where muscle contractions are done with little movement by the body, and are then held static by the muscle.

Julstro Elbow: A multi-functional tool that was specifically designed to help individuals apply pointed pressure to muscle spasms throughout the body.

Julstro Technique: The name of a system of treatments for muscle pains that are caused by repetitive strain injury.

Lactic acid: A natural by-product of muscle action. The body has the mechanism to flush away lactic acid, if it is given sufficient time before more lactic acid is produced.

Lateral: Toward the outer side of the body (i.e.: the arms are lateral to the rib cage).

Ligament: A strong fibrous material that attaches a bone to a bone.

Origin: The point where a muscle or nerve begins. The insertion of a muscle always moves toward the origin.

Lumbar Vertebrae: Spine bones of the low back.

Medial: Toward the center of your body. (I.e.: your chest bone is medial to your shoulder).

Pain referral: The term that describes the condition in which a spasm, or other injury, occurs on one place and is felt in a different place. The area that feels the pain sensation is the pain referral area.

Posterior: Toward the back of your body. (i.e.: your heel is posterior to your toes)

Repetitive strain injury: (RSI) Any muscle injury that is caused by the repeated contraction of a muscle until it either over-contracts or is torn.

Rotator cuff muscles: A group of muscles that enable the arm to rotate at the shoulder joint.

RSI: The abbreviation for Repetitive Strain Injury.

Scapula: (Shoulder Blade) The triangular shaped bone in the upper back. It is the insertion location for many of the muscles that move the arm. This is the area affected by "frozen shoulder".

Shoulder Blade: The common name for the scapula.

Spasm: Involuntary contraction, without release, of a muscle fiber or a group of muscle fibers.

Sternum: (Breastbone) The flat bone in the chest, directly below the chin.

Stiff Neck: When the head cannot move to a full range of motion without pain.

Temporomandibular joint: (TMJ) The hinge joint of the jaw.

Tendon: A strong fibrous material that is the ending portion of the muscle. The tendon inserts onto a bone. Tendons do not have a blood supply, so they heal very slowly.

Tennis Elbow: Also called "briefcase elbow" and many other terms. This condition is caused by the triceps muscle contracting and pulling on the insertion at the elbow. It also prevents the arm from straightening fully without pain in the elbow area.

Thenar muscles: The group name for the muscles that control the thumb.

Thoracic Vertebrae: Spine bones of the mid back.

Trigger Finger: A condition that causes the finger to lock in place when it is bent.

TMJ: See temporomandibular joint.

Trigger points: The name given to spasms, throughout the body, that cause pain to be referred to a different area.

Ulnar bone: The bone of the arm that is easily felt on the same side as the fourth finger (pinky).

Glossary of Muscles

Muscle: [Common nickname] (Muscle Chart #) General location on body

Abdominals: [Abs] (#7) A group of muscles that span the entire lower portion of your anterior trunk.

Biceps: (#2) A muscle that is found on the front of the upper arm.

Deltoid: (#8) Muscle that forms the round part of the upper arm at the shoulder.

Flexors: (#1) A group of separate muscles that work independently to enable your hand to curl into a fist, your fingers to move separately, and your wrist to bend. The tendons of the muscles go through the carpal tunnel.

Erector Spinae: (#10) A group of muscles that move the spine in all directions.

Extensors: (#3, 4, 5) A group of separate muscles that work independently to straighten your fingers and hand from the flexed position, and will pull your hand back (extend).

Gastrocnemius: (gastroc)(#14) Surface calf muscle that pulls the heel up so you can stand on your toes.

Gluteals: (Glutes) Group name for the muscles of the buttocks.

Gluteus Maximus: (#10) (Gluteals) The powerful extensor of the leg, this muscle turns the leg outward.

Gluteus Medius: (#9) (see Gluteals) Located more on the hip than in the buttocks, this muscle is still considered a gluteal muscle. It raises the leg to the side and turns the leg inward.

Gluteus Minimus: (#14, 17) (see Gluteals) Located more on the hip than in the buttocks, this muscle is still considered a gluteal muscle. It raises the leg to the side and turns the leg inward.

Hamstrings: (#13) Muscles in the back part of your thigh. They bend your knee.

Iliopsoas: See "Psoas".

Infraspinatus: (#3) A deep muscle that is located on the lower 2/3 of the shoulder blade.

Latissimus dorsi: (Lats) (#9) Large surface muscle that forms the lower half of the back.

Levator Scapulae: (Levator Scap) (#10) A muscle that goes from the neck to the top of the shoulder blade. It helps you shrug your shoulders.

Opponens Pollicis: Thumb muscle that draws the thumb in toward the palm of the hand.

Pectoralis Major: (#6) The biggest chest muscle.

Pectoralis Minor: (#9) A deep chest muscle that inserts onto the top of the shoulder blade. It helps you shrug your shoulders.

Psoas: (#8, 16) A deep muscle in the abdominal area. It originates on your lumbar vertebrae and inserts into your thighbone.

Quadriceps: (Quads) (#16) Muscles in the front part of your thigh. The "quads" straighten your leg.

Quadratus Lumborum: (QL) (#11) A low back muscle that bends you to the side.

Rhomboid: (#12) Deep muscle that is between the spinal column and the shoulder blade. This muscle pulls the shoulder blades together.

Scalenes: (#1) Muscles of the neck that bring your head down, as if to say "yes". The nerves of the arm pass through these muscles.

SCM (see Sternocleidomastoid)

Serratus Anterior: (#8) A muscle of the chest that is under your arm.

Soleus: (#14) Deep muscle of the calf that works with the gastrocnemius muscle.

Sternalis: (#6) A chest muscle that will cause pain in the chest bone, across the anterior shoulder and down the arm.

Sternocleidomastoid: (#18) A neck muscle that turns your head in the opposite direction.

Subclavius: (#9) Small muscle located directly under your collarbone, near the center of your body.

Supraspinatus: (#10) A deep muscle that is on the top of the shoulder blade. It helps lift your arm.

Tibialis anterior: (T.B.Ant.) (#15) The primary muscle next to the shinbone, it pulls your foot up to lift your toes off the floor.

Trapezius: (Traps) (#6) A large diamond-shaped surface muscle that forms the upper back and curve of the shoulder.

Triceps: (#3, 4) The muscles that are found on the back of the upper arm.

Table of Trigger Point Charts

Table of Muscle Charts

Appendix B – Trigger Point Charts

Trigger Point chart #1
Arms and Hands:
Scalenes and Flexors

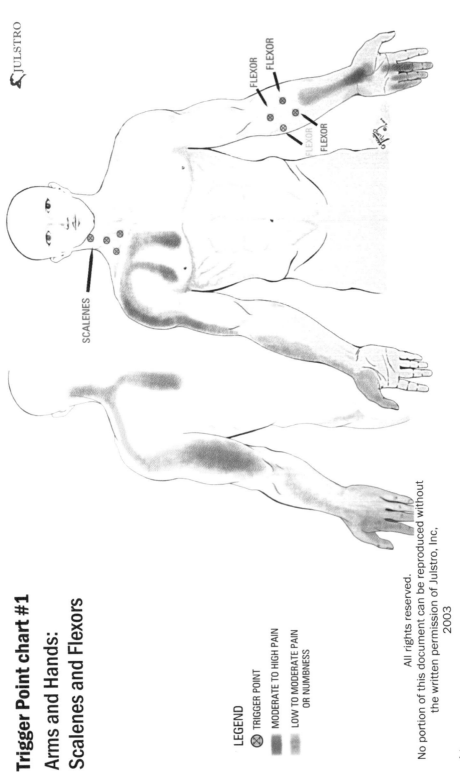

SCALENES

FLEXOR
FLEXOR
FLEXOR
FLEXOR

LEGEND

⊗ TRIGGER POINT

MODERATE TO HIGH PAIN

LOW TO MODERATE PAIN
OR NUMBNESS

Trigger Point chart #2
Shoulder and Arm:
Brachalis, Biceps,
Supinator, Palmaris

LEGEND

⊗ TRIGGER POINT

▬ MODERATE TO HIGH PAIN

▬ LOW TO MODERATE PAIN
OR NUMBNESS

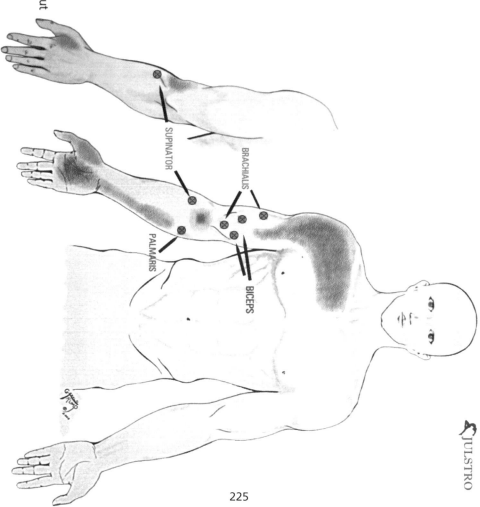

SUPINATOR

BRACHALIS

PALMARIS

BICEPS

JULSTRO

225

Trigger Point chart #3
Shoulder and Arm:
Infraspinatus, Triceps,
Extensor Carpi Ulnaris

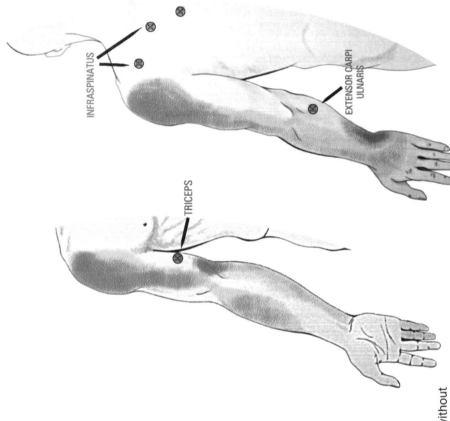

INFRASPINATUS

EXTENSOR CARPI ULNARIS

TRICEPS

LEGEND

⊗ TRIGGER POINT

MODERATE TO HIGH PAIN

LOW TO MODERATE PAIN
OR NUMBNESS

Trigger Point chart # 4
Arms

LEGEND

⊗ TRIGGER POINT

MODERATE TO HIGH PAIN

LOW TO MODERATE PAIN OR NUMBNESS

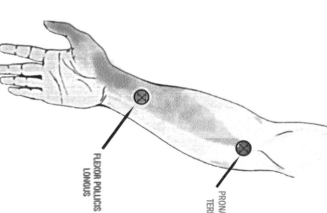

FLEXOR POLLICIS LONGUS

PRONATOR TERES

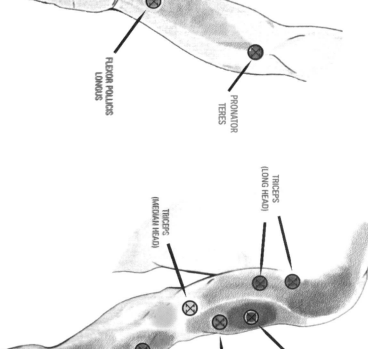

TRICEPS (LONG HEAD)

TRICEPS (MEDIAN HEAD)

TRICEPS (LATERAL HEAD)

TRICEPS (MEDIAN HEAD)

EXTENSOR CARPI RADIALIS LONGUS

𝒮 JULSTRO

Trigger Point chart #5
Forearm and Hand

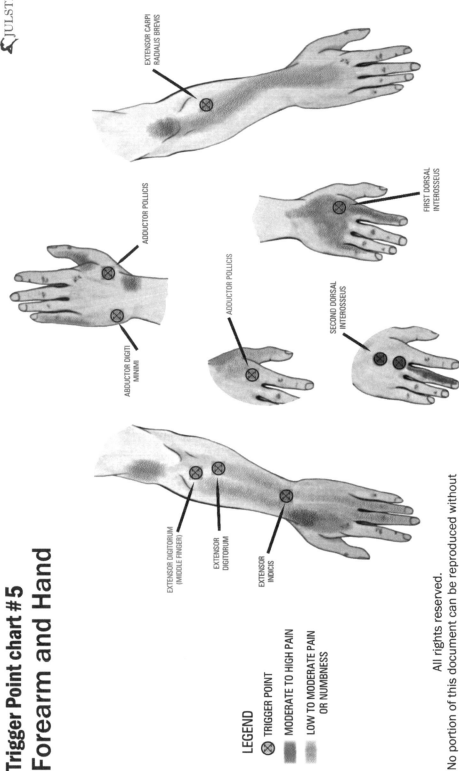

EXTENSOR CARPI RADIALIS BREVIS

FIRST DORSAL INTEROSSEUS

ADDUCTOR POLLICIS

ABDUCTOR DIGITI MINIMI

ADDUCTOR POLLICIS

SECOND DORSAL INTEROSSEUS

EXTENSOR DIGITORUM (MIDDLE FINGER)

EXTENSOR DIGITORUM

EXTENSOR INDICIS

LEGEND

⊗ TRIGGER POINT

MODERATE TO HIGH PAIN

LOW TO MODERATE PAIN OR NUMBNESS

Trigger Point chart # 6
Neck, Shoulder, Chest: Trapezius, Sternalis, Pectoralis

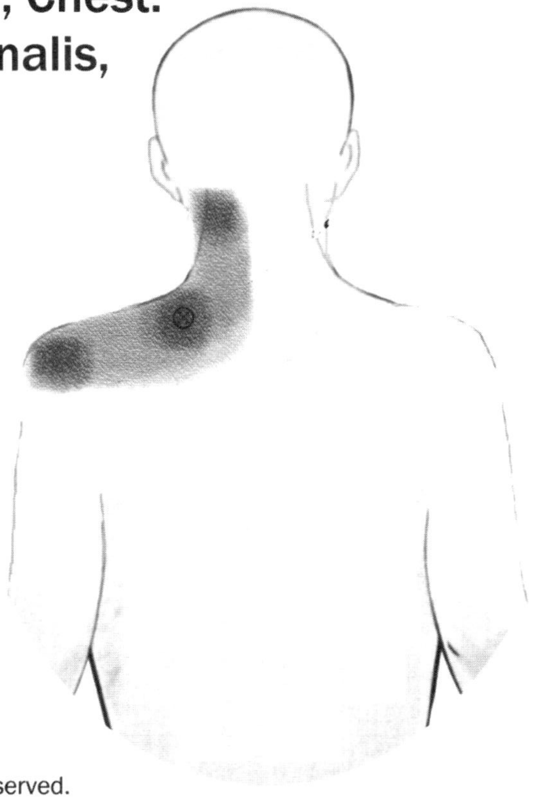

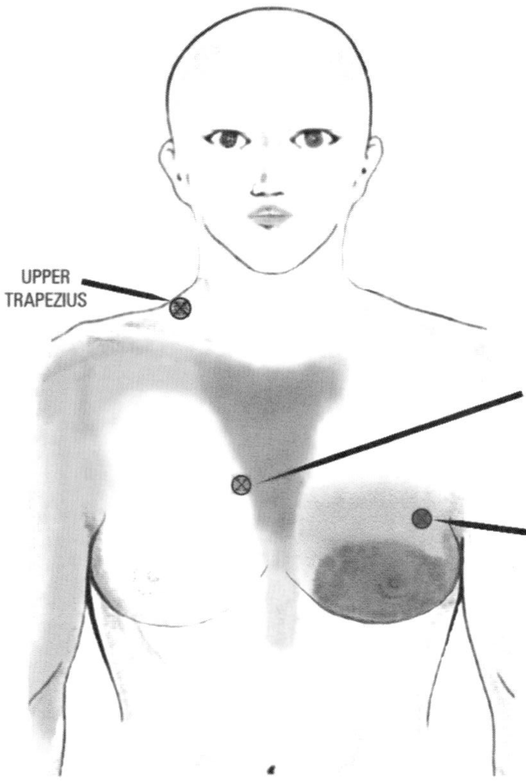

LEGEND

⊗ TRIGGER POINT

MODERATE TO HIGH PAIN

LOW TO MODERATE PAIN OR NUMBNESS

UPPER TRAPEZIUS

STERNALIS

PECTORALIS MAJOR

~JULSTRO

Trigger Point chart #7
Upper Body:
Pectoralis Major,
External Oblique,
Rectus Abdominus,
McBurney's Point

PECTORALIS MAJOR

EXTERNAL OBLIQUE

EXTERNAL OBLIQUE

RECTUS ABDOMINIS

McBURNEY'S POINT

RECTUS ABDOMINIS

LEGEND

⊗ TRIGGER POINT

　　MODERATE TO HIGH PAIN

　　LOW TO MODERATE PAIN
　　OR NUMBNESS

230

Trigger Point chart #8
Upper Body:
Serratus Anterior,
Pectroalis,
Anterior Deltoid,
Iliopsoas (Psoas)

LEGEND

⊗ TRIGGER POINT

MODERATE TO HIGH PAIN

LOW TO MODERATE PAIN
OR NUMBNESS

SERRATUS
ANTERIOR

ILIOPSOAS
(DEEP)

ILIOPSOAS

PECTORALIS
MAJOR

ANTERIOR
DELTOID

JULSTRO

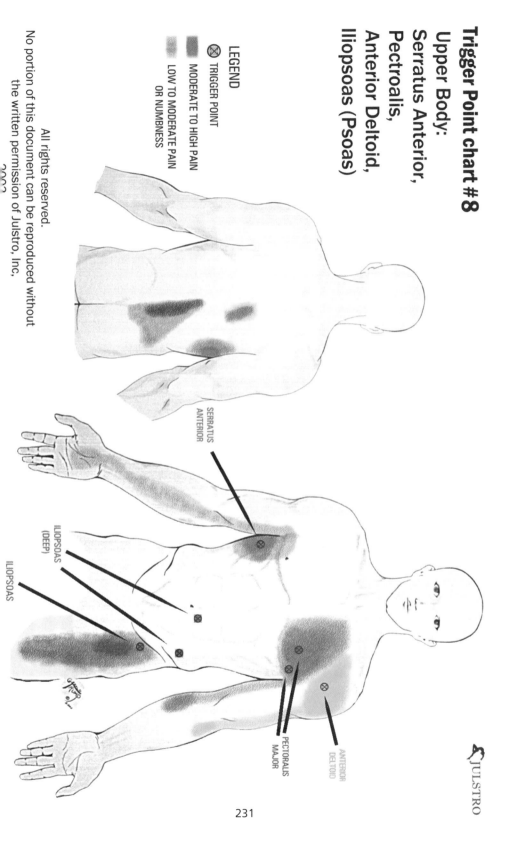

Trigger Point chart #9
Upper Body:
Latissimus, Gluteus,
Ilicostalis, Teres minor,
Subclavius, Pectoralis

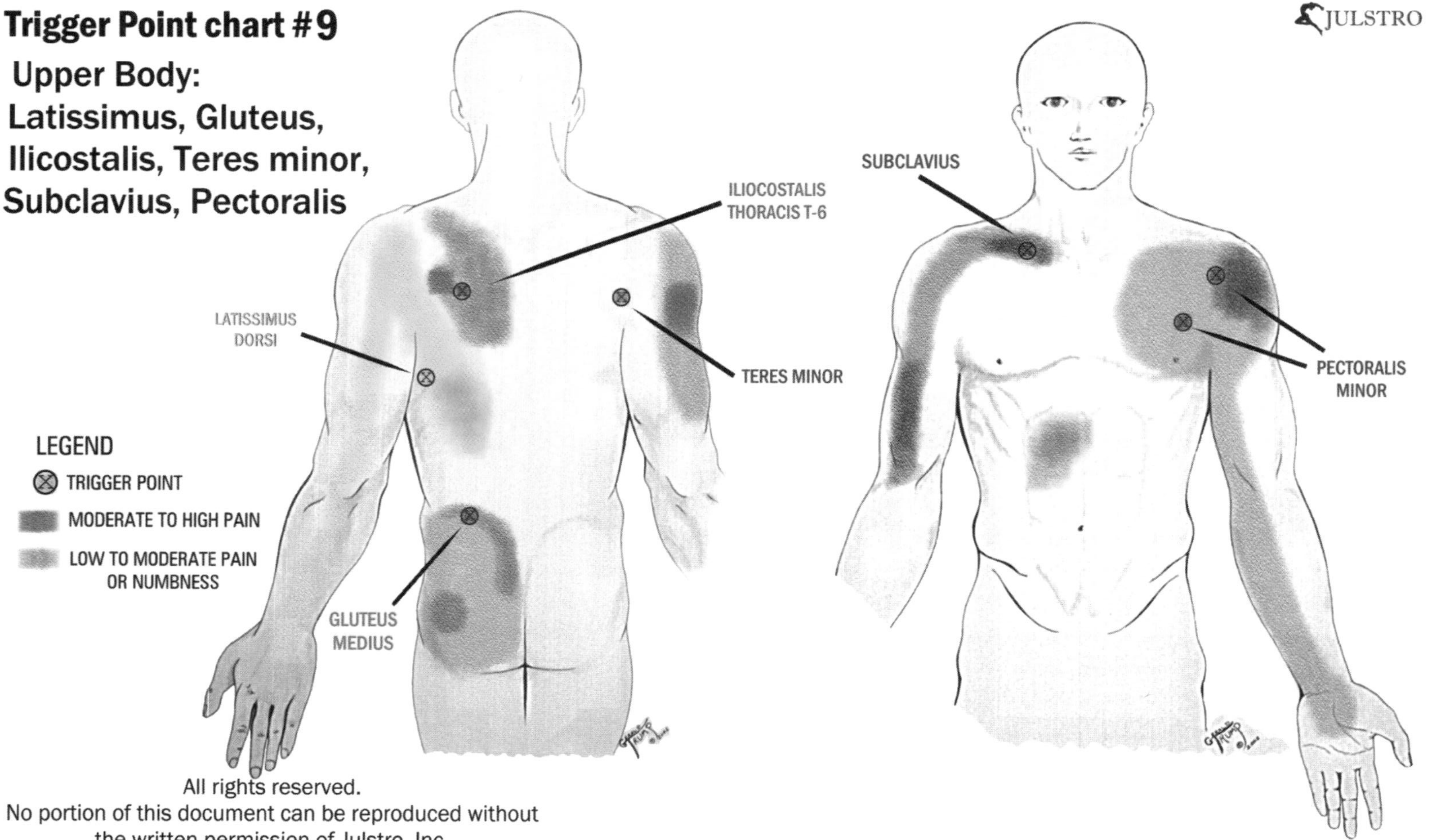

JULSTRO

PECTORALIS MINOR

SUBCLAVIUS

ILIOCOSTALIS THORACIS T-6

TERES MINOR

LATISSIMUS DORSI

GLUTEUS MEDIUS

LEGEND

⊗ TRIGGER POINT

MODERATE TO HIGH PAIN

LOW TO MODERATE PAIN OR NUMBNESS

Trigger Point chart #10
Shoulder, Back and Neck

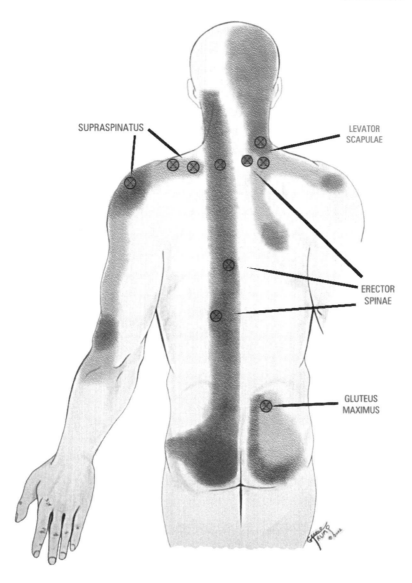

SUPRASPINATUS

LEVATOR SCAPULAE

ERECTOR SPINAE

GLUTEUS MAXIMUS

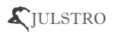

JULSTRO

Trigger Point chart #11
Shoulder and Back:
Trapezius, Deltoid,
Quadratus Lumborum

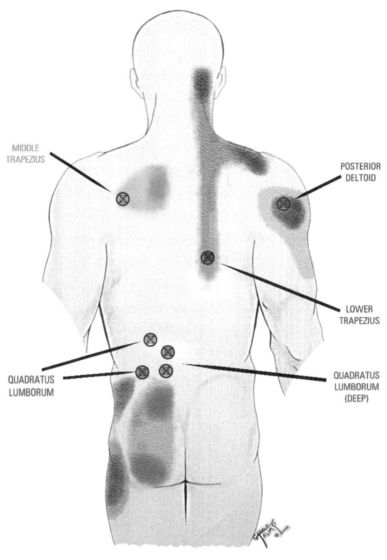

MIDDLE TRAPEZIUS

POSTERIOR DELTOID

LOWER TRAPEZIUS

QUADRATUS LUMBORUM

QUADRATUS LUMBORUM (DEEP)

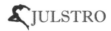

JULSTRO

234   2003

Trigger Point chart #12
Upper Back: Iliocostalis, Rhomboids

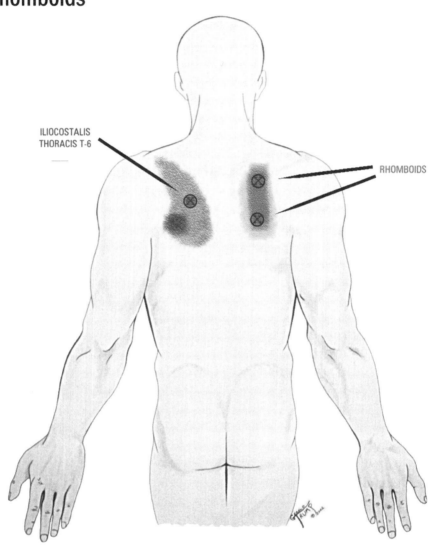

ILIOCOSTALIS THORACIS T-6

RHOMBOIDS

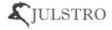 JULSTRO

235

Trigger Point chart #13
Legs, Posterior: Piriformis, Hamstrings

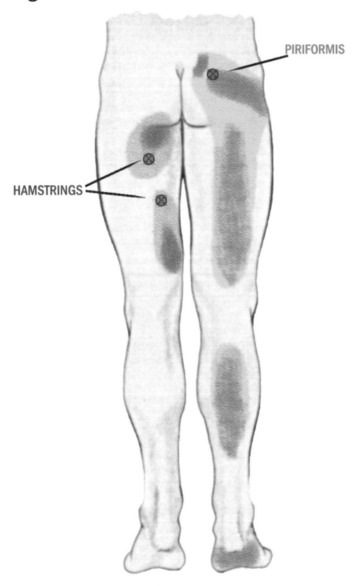

PIRIFORMIS

HAMSTRINGS

JULSTRO

Trigger Point chart #14
Legs, Posterior:

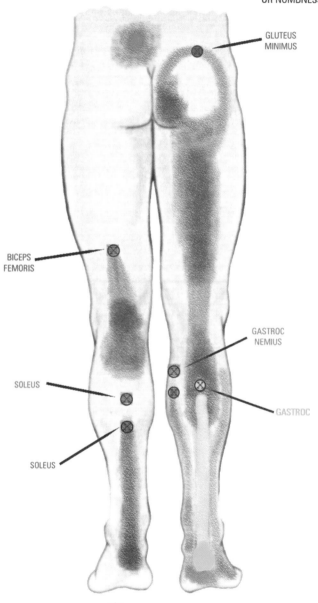

GLUTEUS
MINIMUS

BICEPS
FEMORIS

GASTROC
NEMIUS

SOLEUS

GASTROC

SOLEUS

JULSTRO

Trigger Point chart #15
Leg, Foot(Anterior)

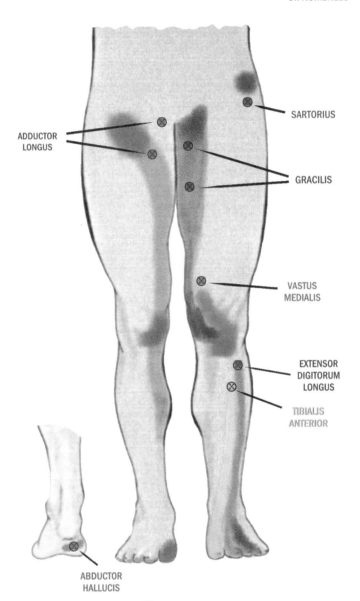

SARTORIUS

ADDUCTOR
LONGUS

GRACILIS

VASTUS
MEDIALIS

EXTENSOR
DIGITORUM
LONGUS

TIBIALIS
ANTERIOR

ABDUCTOR
HALLUCIS

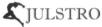

JULSTRO

Trigger Point chart # 16
Iliopsoas (Psoas), Quadricep

LEGEND

⊗ TRIGGER POINT

MODERATE TO HIGH PAIN

LOW TO MODERATE PAIN OR NUMBNESS

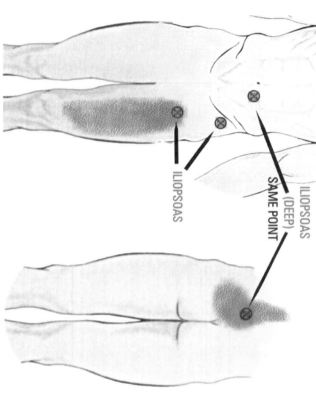

ILIOPSOAS

ILIOPSOAS (DEEP) SAME POINT

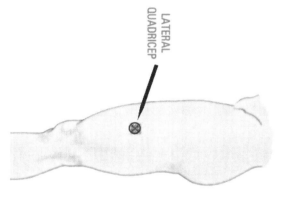

LATERAL QUADRICEP

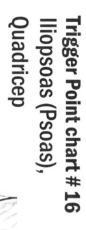

*ʃ*JULSTRO

Trigger Point chart #17
Leg, foot

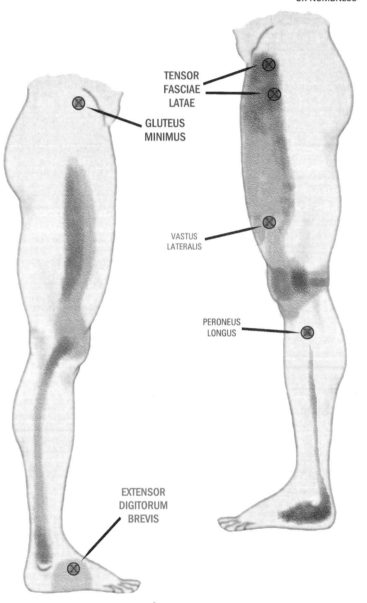

TENSOR
FASCIAE
LATAE

GLUTEUS
MINIMUS

VASTUS
LATERALIS

PERONEUS
LONGUS

EXTENSOR
DIGITORUM
BREVIS

⌇JULSTRO

Trigger Point chart #18
Head, Neck

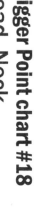

LEGEND

⊗ TRIGGER POINT

MODERATE TO HIGH PAIN

LOW TO MODERATE PAIN
OR NUMBNESS

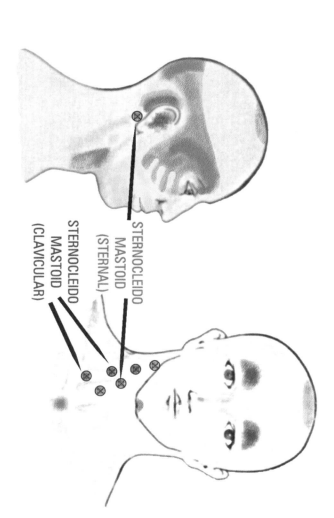

STERNOCLEIDO
MASTOID
(STERNAL)

STERNOCLEIDO
MASTOID
(CLAVICULAR)

JULSTRO

241

Trigger Point chart #19
Head, Face

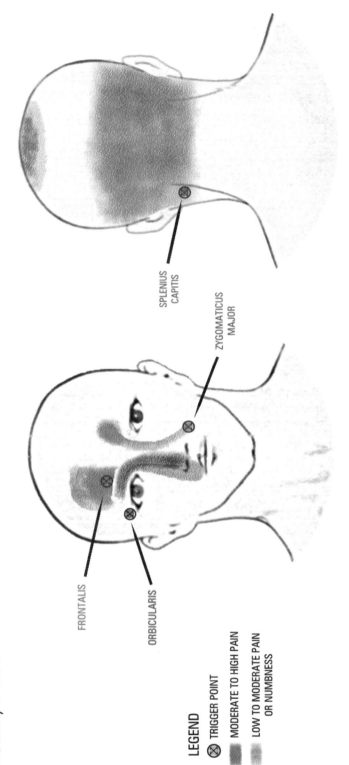

SPLENIUS
CAPITIS

ZYGOMATICUS
MAJOR

FRONTALIS

ORBICULARIS

LEGEND
⊗ TRIGGER POINT

MODERATE TO HIGH PAIN

LOW TO MODERATE PAIN
OR NUMBNESS

Trigger Point chart #20
Head

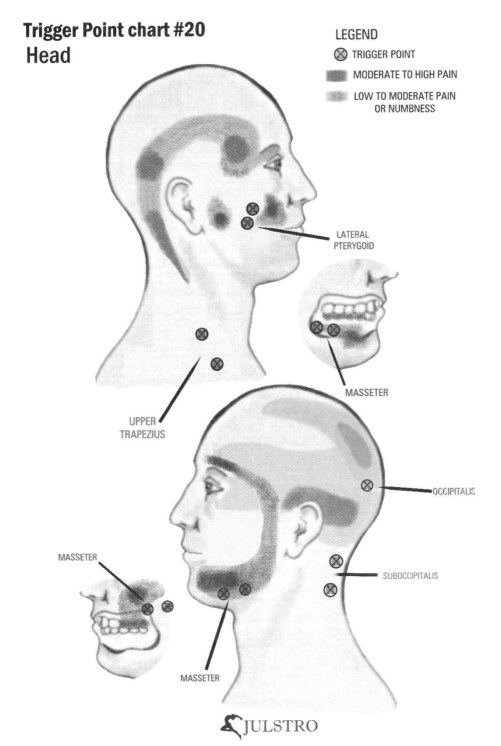

LATERAL
PTERYGOID

MASSETER

UPPER
TRAPEZIUS

OCCIPITALIS

MASSETER

SUBOCCIPITALIS

MASSETER

🦅 JULSTRO

243

Trigger Point chart #21
Face

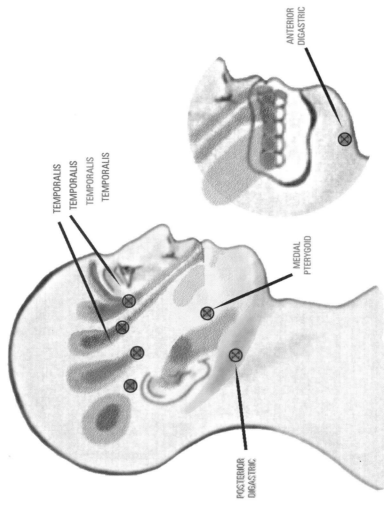

TEMPORALIS
TEMPORALIS
TEMPORALIS
TEMPORALIS

MEDIAL PTERYGOID

POSTERIOR DIGASTRIC

ANTERIOR DIGASTRIC

LEGEND

⊗ TRIGGER POINT

MODERATE TO HIGH PAIN

LOW TO MODERATE PAIN OR NUMBNESS

JULSTRO

Trigger Point chart #22
Hand

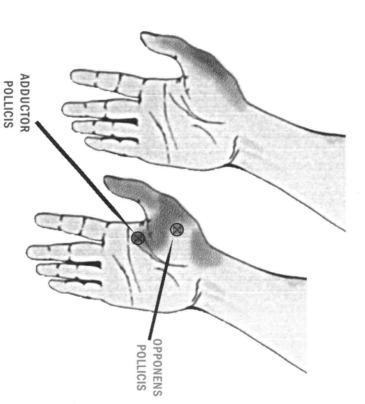

ADDUCTOR POLLICIS

OPPONENS POLLICIS

JULSTRO

245

Appendix C – Muscle Charts

This information is provided as a general reference. If you desire the precise sites of Origin & Insertion, and the technical term for the Action of a muscle, look in a good anatomy textbook.

O – Origin, I – Insertion. A – Action.

Muscle chart #1
Arms and Hands:
Scalenes and Flexors

The following information is provided as a general reference. If you desire the precise sites of Origin & Insertion, and the technical term for the Action of a muscle, look in a good anatomy textbook.

O - is Origin. I - is Insertion. A - is Action

JULSTRO

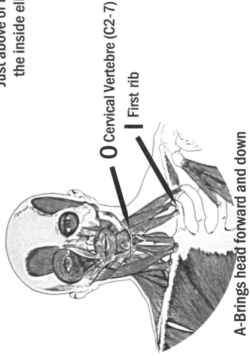

FLEXORS

Just above or below the inside elbow O

At the wrist, hand &-0r fingers

A - Curls fingers into hand and hand towards underside of forearm

SCALENES

O Cervical Vertebre (C2-7)

I First rib

A-Brings head forward and down

Muscle chart #2
Arms and Hands:
Biceps, Supinator, Brachialis, Palmaris

The following information is provided as a general reference. If you desire the precise sites of Origin & Insertion, and the technical term for the Action of a muscle, look in a good anatomy textbook.

O - is Origin. I - is Insertion. A - is Action

𝔍 JULSTRO

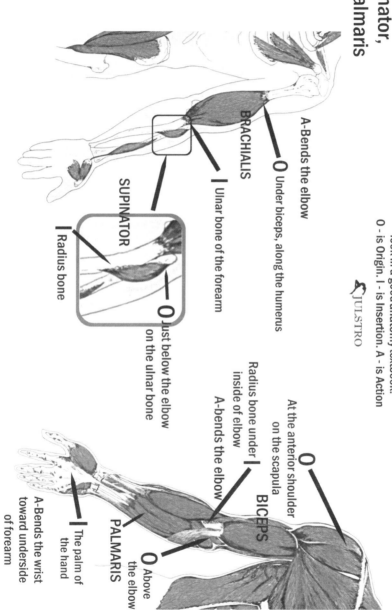

BRACHIALIS

A-Bends the elbow

O Under biceps, along the humerus

I Ulnar bone of the forearm

SUPINATOR

I Radius bone

O Just below the elbow on the ulnar bone

At the anterior shoulder on the scapula

O

Radius bone under inside of elbow I

A-bends the elbow

BICEPS

O Above the elbow

PALMARIS

I The palm of the hand

A-Bends the wrist toward underside of forearm

Muscle chart #3
Arm and Hand:
Infraspinatus,
Triceps,
Extensor Carpi Ulnaris

The following information is provided as a general reference. If you desire the precise sites of Origin & Insertion, and the technical term for the Action of a muscle, look in a good anatomy textbook.

O - is Origin. I - is Insertion. A - is Action

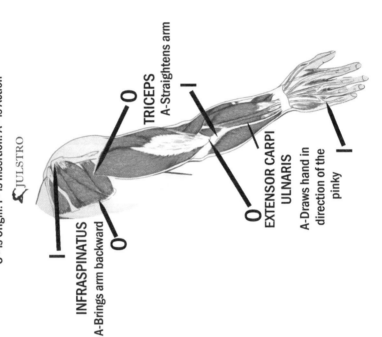

JULSTRO

INFRASPINATUS
A-Brings arm backward

TRICEPS
A-Straightens arm

EXTENSOR CARPI ULNARIS
A-Draws hand in direction of the pinky

Muscle chart #4
Arm and Hand:
Flexor, Triceps,
Pronator, Extensor

The following information is provided as a general reference. If you desire
the precise sites of Origin & Insertion, and the technical term for the Action of a muscle,
look in a good anatomy textbook.
O - is Origin. I - is Insertion. A - is Action

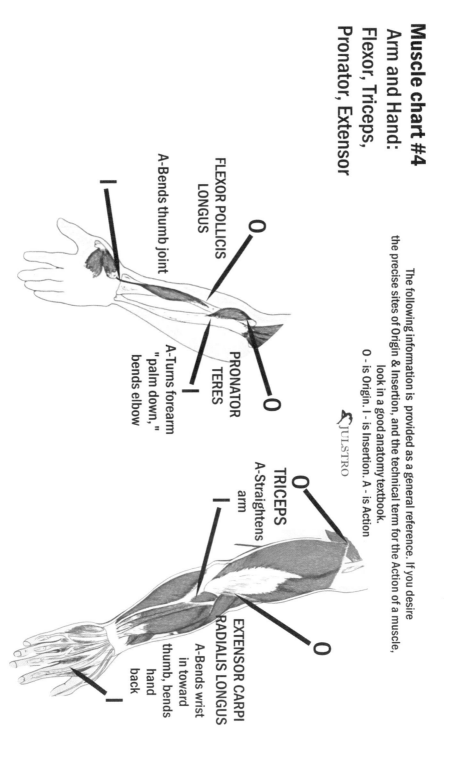

FLEXOR POLLICIS
LONGUS

A-Bends thumb joint

PRONATOR
TERES

A-Turns forearm
"palm down,"
bends elbow

🐬 JULSTRO

TRICEPS
A-Straightens
arm

EXTENSOR CARPI
RADIALIS LONGUS
A-Bends wrist
in toward
thumb, bends
hand
back

Muscle chart #5
Arm and Hand:
Extensors

The following information is provided as a general reference. If you desire the precise sites of Origin & Insertion, and the technical term for the Action of a muscle, look in a good anatomy textbook.

O - is Origin. I - is Insertion. A - is Action

JULSTRO

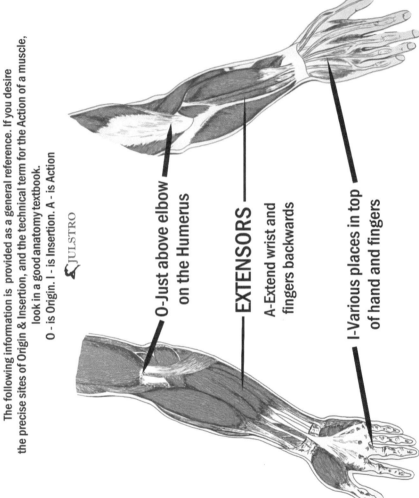

O-Just above elbow on the Humerus

EXTENSORS

A-Extend wrist and fingers backwards

I-Various places in top of hand and fingers

Muscle chart #6
Shoulder, Chest:
Trapezius,
Sternalis,
Pectoralis

The following information is provided as a general reference. If you desire the precise sites of Origin & Insertion, and the technical term for the Action of a muscle, look in a good anatomy textbook.

O - is Origin. I - is Insertion. A - is Action

🦎JULSTRO

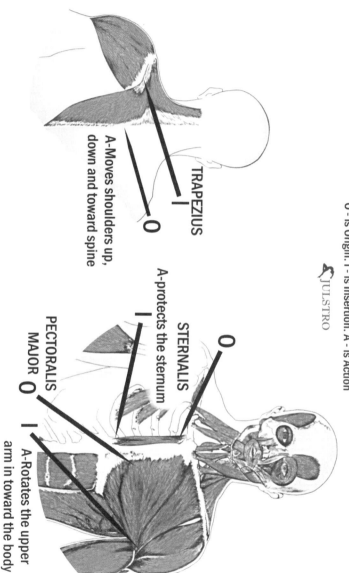

TRAPEZIUS

I

O

A-Moves shoulders up, down and toward spine

STERNALIS

A-protects the sternum

I

O

PECTORALIS MAJOR

O

I

A-Rotates the upper arm in toward the body

253

Muscle chart #7
Abdominals

The following information is provided as a general reference. If you desire the precise sites of Origin & Insertion, and the technical term for the Action of a muscle, look in a good anatomy textbook.

O - is Origin. I - is Insertion. A - is Action

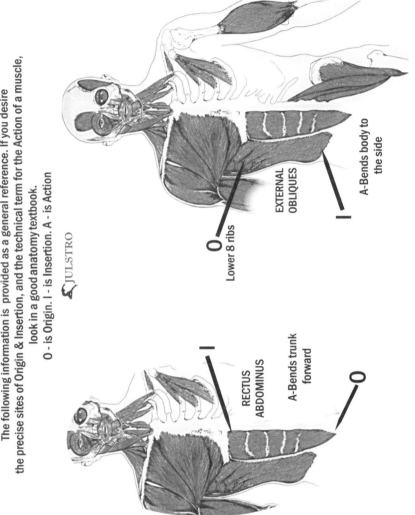

JULSTRO

Lower 8 ribs — O

EXTERNAL OBLIQUES

A-Bends body to the side — I

RECTUS ABDOMINUS

A-Bends trunk forward

I

O

254

Muscle chart #8
Body:
Serratus, Deltoid,
Iliopsoas (Psoas)

The following information is provided as a general reference. If you desire the precise sites of Origin & Insertion, and the technical term for the Action of a muscle, look in a good anatomy textbook.

O - is Origin. I - is Insertion. A - is Action

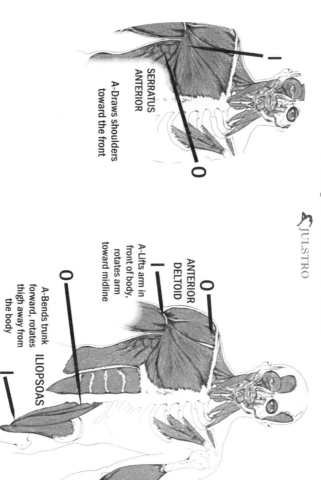

SERRATUS
ANTERIOR

A-Draws shoulders
toward the front

O

I

ANTERIOR
DELTOID

A-Lifts arm in
front of body,
rotates arm
toward midline

O

ILIOPSOAS

A-Bends trunk
forward, rotates
thigh away from
the body

I

O

🐾 JULSTRO

Muscle chart #9
Shoulder, Hip:
Teres, Latissimus,
Subclavius, Pectoralis,
Gluteus Medius

The following information is provided as a general reference. If you desire the precise sites of Origin & Insertion, and the technical term for the Action of a muscle, look in a good anatomy textbook.

O - is Origin. I - is Insertion. A - is Action

JULSTRO

A-Stabilizes collarbone
SUBCLAVIUS O

PECTORALIS MINOR O
A-Draws shoulder forward and down

TERES MINOR O
A-Draws arm back and rotates to the back

GLUTEUS MEDIUS O
A-Lifts leg sideways away from the body and rotates leg toward the midline

LATISSIMUS DORSI O
A-Draws arm down and rotates in

Muscle chart #10
Shoulder, Back, Hip:

The following information is provided as a general reference. If you desire the precise sites of Origin & Insertion, and the technical term for the Action of a muscle, look in a good anatomy textbook.

O - is Origin. I - is Insertion. A - is Action

JULSTRO

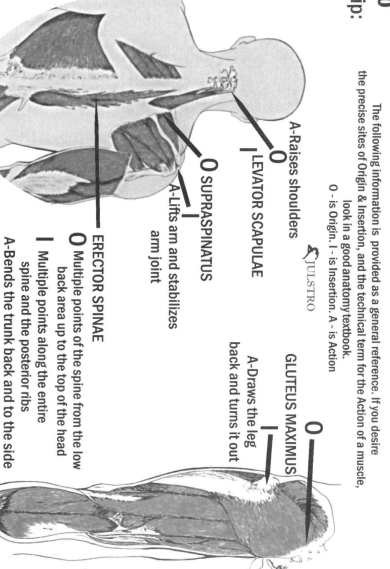

A-Raises shoulders

O

I LEVATOR SCAPULAE

O SUPRASPINATUS
I
A-Lifts arm and stabilizes
arm joint

ERECTOR SPINAE

O Multiple points of the spine from the low
back area up to the top of the head

I Multiple points along the entire
spine and the posterior ribs

A-Bends the trunk back and to the side

O

GLUTEUS MAXIMUS
I
A-Draws the leg
back and turns it out

257

Muscle chart #11
Low Back:
Quadratus Lumborum

The following information is provided as a general reference. If you desire the precise sites of Origin & Insertion, and the technical term for the Action of a muscle, look in a good anatomy textbook.

O - is Origin. I - is Insertion. A - is Action

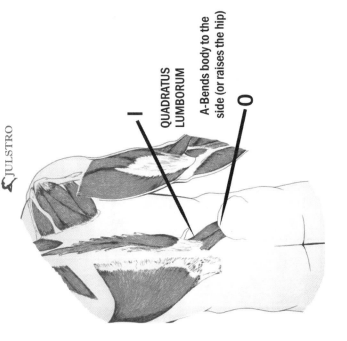

𝓛JULSTRO

I

QUADRATUS LUMBORUM

A-Bends body to the side (or raises the hip)

O

Muscle chart #12

Back:
Rhomboids

The following information is provided as a general reference. If you desire
the precise sites of Origin & Insertion, and the technical term for the Action of a muscle,
look in a good anatomy textbook.
O - is Origin. I - is Insertion. A - is Action

🐾 JULSTRO

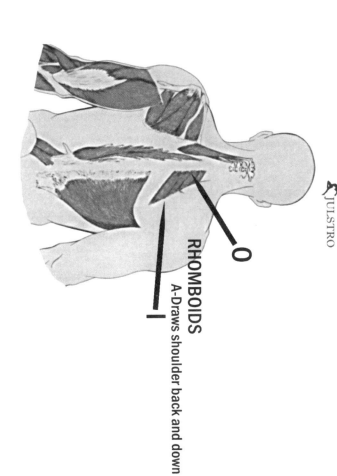

O

RHOMBOIDS
A-Draws shoulder back and down

I

Muscle chart #13
Hamstrings, Piriformis

The following information is provided as a general reference. If you desire the precise sites of Origin & Insertion, and the technical term for the Action of a muscle, look in a good anatomy textbook.

O - is Origin. I - is Insertion. A - is Action

JULSTRO

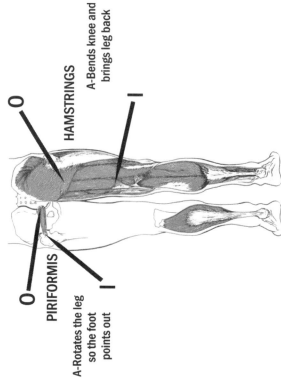

HAMSTRINGS

A-Bends knee and brings leg back

PIRIFORMIS

A-Rotates the leg so the foot points out

Muscle chart #14
Leg:
Gluteus, Soleus, Gastroc

The following information is provided as a general reference. If you desire the precise sites of Origin & Insertion, and the technical term for the Action of a muscle, look in a good anatomy textbook.

O - is Origin. I - is Insertion. A - is Action

JULSTRO

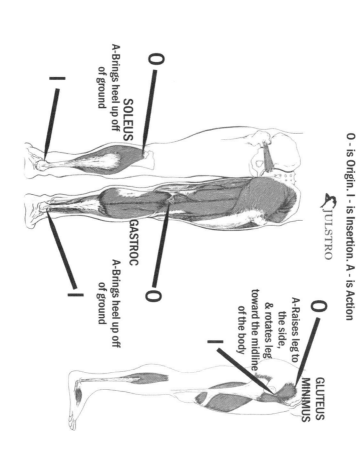

SOLEUS
A-Brings heel up off of ground

GASTROC
A-Brings heel up off of ground

GLUTEUS MINIMUS
A-Raises leg to the side, & rotates leg toward the midline of the body

Muscle chart #15
Leg. Foot

The following information is provided as a general reference. If you desire the precise sites of Origin & Insertion, and the technical term for the Action of a muscle, look in a good anatomy textbook.

O - is Origin. I - is Insertion. A - is Action

𝕁JULSTRO

GRACILIS
A-Bends knee and rotates knee toward centerline of body

SATORIUS
A-Brings leg into "crossed leg" squatting position

ADDUCTOR LONGUS
A-Bends the knee forward, flexes the hip

EXTENSOR DIGITORUM
A-Pulls up on toes and assists in raising front of foot off the floor

ABDUCTOR HALLICUS
A-Curls foot by drawing big toe in toward arch

Muscle chart #16

Leg:
Iliopsoas (Psoas),
Quadriceps

The following information is provided as a general reference. If you desire the precise sites of Origin & Insertion, and the technical term for the Action of a muscle, look in a good anatomy textbook.

O - is Origin. I - is Insertion. A - is Action

🐾 JULSTRO

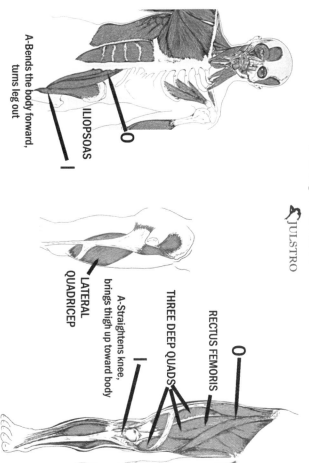

ILIOPSOAS

O

I

A-Bends the body forward, turns leg out

LATERAL
QUADRICEP

THREE DEEP QUADS

RECTUS FEMORIS

O

I

A-Straightens knee, brings thigh up toward body

Muscle chart #17
Leg, Foot:
Gluteus Minimus,
Tensor Fasciae Latae,
Peroneus Longus,
Extensor Digitorum Brevis

The following information is provided as a general reference. If you desire the precise sites of Origin & Insertion, and the technical term for the Action of a muscle, look in a good anatomy textbook.

O - is Origin. I - is Insertion. A - is Action

JULSTRO

O TENSOR FASCIAE LATAE

A-Stabilizes the knee, assists in bending knee

I

O PERONEUS LONGUS

A-Lifts outside edge of foot off the floor

I

O GLUTEUS MINIMUS

A-Draws leg away from the body; rotates thigh toward center

I

EXTENSOR DIGITORUM BREVIS

O

I A-Lifts toes off the floor

Muscle chart #18
Neck

The following information is provided as a general reference. If you desire the precise sites of Origin & Insertion, and the technical term for the Action of a muscle, look in a good anatomy textbook.

O - is Origin. I - is Insertion. A - is Action

JULSTRO

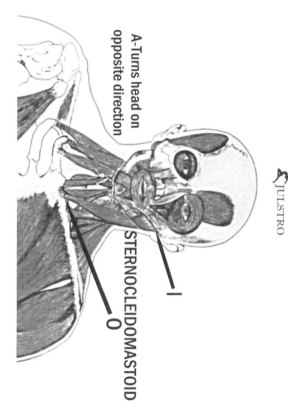

A-Turns head on opposite direction

STERNOCLEIDOMASTOID

I

O

Makai Press
PUBLICATIONS
79 Church Street, Nanuet, NY 10954
Julstro, Inc. product information
Telephone: (845) 268-2021
Toll free: 1-866- SELF TREAT (1-866-735-3873)
e-mail: orders@julstro.com WEBSITE: www.julstro.com

Products

E-BOOKS

The "Pain-Free" series of e-books are conveniently sent via email to your computer, with links to the full color Trigger Point Charts, and informative Muscle Charts that guides each Julstro self-treatment.

	Price
The Pain-Free Triathlete	**$39.95**
The Pain-Free Runner	**$12.95**
The Pain-Free Swimmer	**$12.95**

BOOKS –

The Pain-Free Runner	**$19.95**
Shipping	$8.50
(add $2.00 for each additional)	

Carpal Tunnel Syndrome:

What you don't know CAN hurt you	**$9.95**
Shipping	$7.50
(add $2.00 for each additional)	
The Pain-Free Triathlete	**$46.95**
Shipping	$10.50
(add $3.00 for each additional)	

TOOLS –

The TP Massage Ball w/Video	**$24.99**
Shipping	$6.85
The TP Massage Foot Baller Set	**$49.99**
Shipping	$8.75
The Complete TP Massage Set	**$69.99**
Shipping	$8.75

VIDEO –

The Julstro self-treatment Video System
For Carpal Tunnel Syndrome

And hand and wrist pain	**$149.95**
Shipping	$15.00
(International orders add $15.00)	

ORDER FORM IS ON THE BACK OF THIS PAGE:
Mail to the address above.

ORDER FORM

The Pain-Free Runner e-book **$12.95** quantity [ ] total [ ]

The Pain-Free Swimmer e-book **$12.95** quantity [ ] total [ ]

The Pain-Free Triathlete e-book **$39.95** quantity [ ] total [ ]

The Pain-Free Runner book **$19.95** quantity [ ] total [ ]

The Pain-Free Triathlete book **$46.95** quantity [ ] total [ ]

Carpal Tunnel Syndrome book **$10.95** quantity [ ] total [ ]

The TP Massage Ball w/Video **$24.99** quantity [ ] total [ ]

The TP Massage Foot Baller Set **$49.99** quantity [ ] total [ ]

The Complete TP Massage Set **$69.99** quantity [ ] total [ ]

Self Treatment Carpal Tunnel
Video System **$149.95** quantity [ ] total [ ]

Add applicable shipping [ ]

Sub total [ ]

(New York residents add 7.9% sales tax) [ ]

Total Order [ ]

Payment: Check ❏   Visa ❏   Master Card ❏   Amex ❏

Shipping and billing address: _____

Name (as it appears on the card): _____

Company (or C/O) _____

Address: _____

| City | State | Zip | Country |

Credit Card number: _____

Expiration Date: _____

Month / Year

Signature: _____